DECARB DIET

....
GUIDE
to a
LOW CARB
Lifestyle

The
DECARB DIET

....

GUIDE
to a
LOW CARB
Lifestyle

Dr Howard Rybko

The right of Dr Howard Rybko to be identified as the author of this work has been asserted. No part of this publication my may be reproduced, stored or transmitted, in any form or by any means, without prior written permission of the publisher. All rights reserved.

2nd CreateSpace Edition January 2015
© Dr Howard Rybko
ISBN-13: 978-1507501672

Originally Published by Porcupine Press - South Africa

howard@decarbdiet.com
www.decarbdiet.com
Cover and text by Wim Rheeder

CONTENTS

INTRODUCTION — 13

The Beginning — 14
About the Decarb Diet and Lifestyle Program — 17
Principles of the Decarb Diet — 20
Why You Need to Avoid Carbs — 21
Why You Have to Balance Your Omega's — 22
Why You Don't Have to Exercise – But You Should Anyway — 24
Assess Yourself — 25

WHAT — 26

PREPARATION — 28
Measure and Record Your Baselines — 29
Set Your Personal Goals — 32
Prepare Your Kitchen — 33
Learn to Read Labels — 35
Supermarket Survival — 40
Surviving Eating Out — 43
Recommended Supplements — 44
Stress — 49

STRIKE — 53
Forbidden Foods — 56
What Else to Watch Out For — 58
Allowed Foods — 60
Some Examples of Low Carb Meals — 63
Recording Your Progress — 65

STABILISATION	66
Plateau Busting	69
Using a Glucose Meter	73

WHY — 75

What is Carbohydrate Resistance?	76
Is There Such a Thing as Carbohydrate Addiction?	79
Eating Too Much? You Fat Lazy Thing!	81
Silly Idea: Calories In = Calories Out	83
Sugar: Sweet Suicide	86
Fructose is a Poison	92
Ketones – Primary Fuel	96
More About Insulin	97
Why You Need to Know About AGEs	98
You Don't Need Carbs to Survive	99
The Worldwide Diabetes Epidemic	101
Achieving Omega Balance is Critical for Your Health	103
Human Origins and the Paleo Diet	105
Exercise to Lose Weight? It's Not Going to Work!	110
The Hidden Dangers of Sitting	113
Away From Health – Dietary Goals for the United States	115
Sports Drinks, Energy Drinks – Just Say No!	116
Keto-Adaptation For Weekend Warriors	118
Keto-Adaptation Time	120
Carbo-Loading is Old Technology	122
My Story	124
Further Reading	127

TOOLKIT 129

GUIDES AND CHARTS 130

General Carb Guide 130

Carbs in Common Vegetables 137

Omega Food Balance Scores 139

Blood Sugar Levels 144

RECIPES 146

Low Carb, High Fat Breakfasts 146

Lunch 154

Dinner 161

SAMPLE JOURNALS 167

Daily Journal 167

Weight Journal 169

Exercise Journal 171

Body Measurements Journal 173

Blood Sugar Journal 175

ENDNOTES 177

For my beloved wife Gail, who is always by my side.

For our children, our life:

Caitlin (my philosopher),

Paige (my editor), and

Gabriel (my sounding board & culinary advisor).

To Professor Tim Noakes,

who asked me to 'Help spread the word'.

I'm spreading it, Prof.

WHAT SOME DIETERS HAVE TO SAY ABOUT DECARB

'Decarb changed my life.' Craig, 24

'30 kg and counting …' Anita, 60

'My sugar is brilliant, I'm feeling so much better and have so much more energy.' Marcie, 55

'I dropped 16 kg six months ago and it has stayed off … Decarb is the only diet that has ever worked for me.' Gary, 41

'Halved my insulin requirements and doubled my energy levels!' Shaun, 38

'Bye-bye to my blood pressure pills and 10 kg to boot.' Michelle, 51

'After 5 weeks on Decarb, my wife hugged me and said, "What's this lump?" I laughed. "It's a rib you haven't felt in 15 years!"' Jonathan, 48

'The How To guides made it easy for me to get into and it seems to be working, I lost 3 kilos in the first week!' Lynette, 44

'When I wake up in the mornings my eyes pop open and I have so much energy that I jump out of bed.' Jill, 53

DISCLAIMER

This program advocates a low carbohydrate, high fat diet. It also drives the reduction of omega-6 fatty acid intake, along with an increase of omega-3's, so as to attain a tissue balance of these two fatty acids that is as close as 1:1 as possible. Normalisation of vitamin D levels is also advocated along with vitamin D supplementation.

The program advocates the eating of certain protein and dairy products. As a result there may also be an increase in the protein intake of a person following this diet.

These types of animal products contain relatively higher levels of saturated fats, which some parts of the medical and nutritional community consider to be unhealthy for your heart and blood vessels. (Most of these same authorities also consider cholesterol-lowering drugs to be good for you.)

In line with a growing number of medical and scientific sources, I do not consider saturated fats to be harmful to our health, especially since we have been eating them in copious amounts for the past few million years without obvious harm, until the aforementioned authorities decided that they were bad for us. I do however consider restoration of the balance between the omega-6 and omega-3 fatty acids as well as normal vitamin D levels to be of critical importance for good health and normal body weight.

Although millions of people have safely and successfully transformed their lives by converting to a low carbohydrate diet there are some individuals who should approach this kind of diet with caution. The types of patients mentioned below should consult their medical professionals before embarking on the program. Those potentially at risk include:

- *diabetic patients taking blood-sugar-lowering medication*
- *patients with high blood pressure and on medication for this (because the diet may lower your blood pressure and your dose will need to be adjusted)*
- *kidney disease patients (although this program is **not** a high protein diet)*
- *patients suffering from gallstones or gall bladder attacks*

- any patient with a history of cardiovascular disease, cancer or liver disease.

Efficacy

While the Decarb Diet should work for anyone who follows it, there may be the occasional individual for whom the diet does not work. Nevertheless the diet will most assuredly work for the majority who follow it. There are, however, differing levels of achievable leanness, based on individual make-up and historical eating patterns. Thus in certain cases, some individuals may find that the diet does not achieve the ultimate leanness that they aspire to.

TALK TO ME

Send me an email: readers@decarbdiet.com

Facebook: facebook.com/decarbdiet

Visit the website: decarbdiet.com

HOW TO USE THIS BOOK

There are two main sections in this book.

- **What – What You Have to Do, and**
- **Why – The Science Behind the Diet.**

To follow the diet and benefit from the program, all you need to do is read 'What'. If you would like to understand why the program is structured the way it is, read 'Why'.

A great deal of research and planning has gone into the development of this Decarb Diet, which differs from similar diets in that it also focuses on what is known as Omega Balance. All the background and research is explained in an easy-to-follow way in the Why section.

You can become lean and rescue your health without ever looking at the Why section. However, read it if you want to understand more. You can also dip into it from time to time as you feel the need to know more.

This image **READ MORE** indicates that there is a section further on in the book that has more detailed information about the topic under discussion.

The Introduction gives you a brief overview of the program and the theory behind it. The last section of the book, Toolkit, is a useful reference section. It contains various lists and charts, recipes, and sample journal pages.

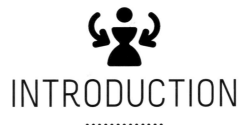

INTRODUCTION

The Decarb Diet was inspired by my wife, who shoved a news-clipping under my disinterested nose. There was a picture of a slim and beaming Professor Tim Noakes, holding a plate of forbidden foods like cheese, cream and red meat. The text explained how much weight he had lost after he turned his back on years of carbohydrate evangelism and embraced a high fat diet.

With a scant six weeks to go to my 15th Argus Cycle Tour, I was in my usual state of semi-readiness. My training was on track but I lacked the willpower to eat less in conjunction with the harder training. Knowing full well that I would, as usual, start the race at least seven kilograms too heavy, I decided that I had nothing to lose. From the moment I put that article down, I stopped eating carbs and switched to a high fat diet.

Magically, it worked. Even though I ate as much as I wanted over the next four weeks, five kilograms melted from my mid-section and I arrived in Cape Town wearing jeans that had hung in my cupboard for almost 20 years!

I hope that you will have the courage to follow the same route that I took, and that the additional guidance and information contained in this book will make it easier for you to travel the road to good health and a body that looks and functions the way it was designed to do.

Try the Decarb Diet for two or three weeks and you will not believe how different you will feel as your body switches to burning the fuel it was designed to run on.

Good luck!

THE BEGINNING

The initial ideas behind the Decarb Diet came out of the work of Professor Tim Noakes, the books of Gary Taubes and the famous video *Sugar: The Bitter Truth* by Professor Robert Lustig. What they had to say highlighted the role of sugar and refined carbohydrates in the decline of health worldwide over the past century. These books were soon followed by a library of others, some of which are listed in the 'Further Reading' section at the end of the WHY section.

We humans were never designed to eat sugars in anything but tiny quantities. We originated in a world where sugar was so rare that we became hardwired to seek out and consume as much sugar or sweet stuff as we could get our hands on.

Consider the lab rats that were purposely addicted to cocaine. When given a choice between feeding their cocaine habit or eating some sweet stuff, guess which they chose? They went for the sweet stuff, every time.[1]

We are programmed to seek sweetness in a similar way to those lab rats.

This fact is totally lost on the average Joe, who is happy to bombard his system with up to 35 teaspoons of sugar every day. The average sugar intake per person in the USA in 2005 was 120 lbs. per year.[2] This translates into almost 150 grams (or 35 teaspoons) of sugar a day. It is hardly surprising that so many people's systems begin to buckle under the load and the inevitable health consequences of diabetes and others maladies rear their heads.

As I dug deeper and did more research I begin to see things more clearly. We humans existed largely unchanged for over two hundred thousand years. Over this period, our diet and activities remained unchanged.

It is only in the past few thousand years, with the advent of agriculture, that these habits, practised for almost ten thousand generations, began to change. In evolutionary terms these changes have happened much too fast for our bodies to adapt to. As a result many of us are still unable to tolerate carbohydrates in any significant quantity.

In addition to our intolerance of carbs, there are two other consequences which I believe are of major significance to our health.

1. Almost all of us are deficient in omega-3 fatty acids, because these essential fatty acids have been systematically removed from our food supply.
2. Almost all of us are deficient in vitamin D, since we no longer spend much time in the sun.

The combination of these two deficiencies with the sugar and carbohydrate tsunami makes us sick and sad.

Your Missing Omega-3's and Vitamin D

The Decarb Diet advocates (as do many other low carb diets) a low carb lifestyle. Adoption of this kind of diet automatically results in higher fat consumption, which predictably results in weight loss and improved health.

However, there is still a problem. In order to be really healthy and not just lean, we need to add the other two missing ingredients to our diet. When we do, our health improves, inflammation decreases and general well-being results.

Omega-3 Deficiency

The deficiency of omega-3's in our diet has been implicated in the development of a number of inflammatory conditions, including arthritis, asthma and psychiatric disorders. Omega-3 deficiency may also increase a tendency to develop cancer and heart disease.

When your body is deficient in omega-3, your omega-6 to omega-3 ratio goes out of balance and your general inflammation levels rise.

It is estimated that the average omega-6 to omega-3 ratio in city dwellers is about 15:1. Compare this to our ancestors whose ratios were close to 1:1.

An effort to increase your levels of omega-3 fatty acids is an integral part of the Decarb Diet. The program encourages you to eat more fish and more greens, and to take omega-3 supplements. These measures will speed up your weight reduction efforts and will greatly enhance your general health.

The Global Vitamin D Deficiency

The other missing ingredient is vitamin D. (In fact, vitamin D is actually a hormone and not a vitamin.) It is generally believed that up to 80% of the American and European population is deficient in vitamin D.[3]

The current mantra of 'sun phobia', whereby the medical establishment has demonised exposure to the sun, has resulted in most people either avoiding the sun altogether or else wearing sunscreen whenever they are exposed to sunlight. To make matters worse, our clothes also limit our body's exposure to the sun.

Thus even in sunny climes, where natural maintenance of normal vitamin D levels would be possible, many avoid sun exposure and become deficient in this vital hormone.

What are the consequences of vitamin D deficiency? Here is a short list:

- Depression (especially seasonal)
- Increased susceptibility to breast cancer
- Weight gain and increased insulin resistance

Our ancestors, who had a limited choice of clothing options, were exposed to sunlight whenever it was sunny. As a result many processes in the body depend on high levels of vitamin D.

The Decarb Diet Program will strive to ensure that your vitamin D levels are returned to normal as soon as possible.

ABOUT THE DECARB DIET AND LIFESTYLE PROGRAM

This program is not really a diet. It is a healthy eating program that will enhance your life, by reducing your carbohydrate intake and balancing your omega-3 intake.

It will:

- Greatly decrease your chances of developing cancer, heart problems or Alzheimer's
- Restore your normal hormonal functions and reduce your chances of getting diabetes
- Raise your energy levels
- Speed up your metabolism
- Slow down your ageing processes
- Add some extra years to your lifespan

And yes, you will also lose weight.

Program Basics

This program is based on a low carb, high fat diet. It is guided by proven medical research and is based on the natural diet our ancestors thrived on, which comprised mainly animal fat, protein, greens and some vegetables.[4]

The diet aims to help you to:

- Remove or greatly reduce the carbs in your diet
- Restore your normal balance of essential fatty acids

Program Background

An oversupply of sugar and refined carbs in our diet, combined with an abundance of omega-6 fats, has had devastating effects on our health.

We are like frogs in a pot of water on the stove, complacent and comfortable as the water slowly boils. In a similar way, our health and the health of our society have been slowly degenerating. Each year, we get a little sicker and little fatter.

This state of affairs suits everyone, except us. As we eat more junk, we get sicker and fuel the world's greatest industries in a torrent of cash that helps to keep the world's governments afloat. Our degeneration is driven by a complex of mega industries:

- A global food industry that manufactures mountains of deadly foodstuffs, designed for long shelf life and formulated to trigger our hardwired unhealthy behaviour to eat more sweet stuff
- A media and marketing machine that force-feeds the junk to us and our children, using every possible medium and subterfuge imaginable
- A medical industry that peddles expensive cures for the diseases we develop and medical insurance against the diseases we are certain to develop as we consume more of our poisonous food supply
- Governments and health agencies that spend so much energy on disease and so little on disease prevention

Program Benefits

This program is designed to stop you eating carbohydrates so that you can stabilise your blood sugar levels and thus control your weight and optimise your general health.

You will also learn that weight control is more about your health than about how you look. If you are overweight, you are engaged in a game of life or death, your life and your death. (New research shows that being moderately overweight can reduce your lifespan by up to three years. Severe obesity can shorten a person's life by up to ten years.) [5]

In addition to reducing your weight, this program will help you dodge the killer diseases of diabetes, heart attacks, cancer and Alzheimer's.

If you make some personal sacrifices and follow the Three Phases of the Decarb Diet, you will:

- Never be hungry
- Become lean without much effort
- Improve your health
- Drop your weight
- Raise your energy levels
- Brighten your outlook on life
- Prevent premature ageing

You won't:

- Count calories
- Be hungry
- Have to exercise to lose weight

PRINCIPLES OF THE DECARB DIET

These are the principles upon which the diet is based. I wish I had known them years ago.

- *Being overweight has nothing to do with overeating, laziness or lack of exercise.*
- *We get fat by eating carbohydrates, which make us fat by stimulating insulin.*
- *Eating fat does not make us fat, nor does it cause heart disease.*
- *The carbohydrates in our diet are primarily responsible for obesity, diabetes, heart disease, cancer and Alzheimer's.*
- *The carbohydrates in our diet make us hungry and decrease our energy levels.*
- *Sugar and high fructose corn syrup are deadly for our health.*
- *Counting calories is ridiculous and eating excess good calories will no more make us grow fatter than it will make us grow taller. Good calories are calories that do not come from sugar or refined carbohydrates.*
- *It is impossible to lose weight by exercising more; however, exercise is vital for wellness and maintaining the insulin sensitivity of our muscles.*
- *It is essential that we maintain a correct omega-6 to omega-3 balance in our bodies by decreasing our omega-6 intake and increasing our omega-3 intake. By achieving a proper omega balance we enhance our insulin sensitivity, increase our metabolic rates, reduce overall inflammation and limit our tendencies towards heart disease, neurological disorders and cancer.*
- *Most of us are vitamin D deficient and need vitamin D supplementation to restore normal levels. Normal vitamin D levels are essential for our mental well-being as well as for maintaining insulin sensitivity and resistance to cancer and infections.*

WHY YOU NEED TO AVOID CARBS

The Decarb program promotes the removal of sugar and refined carbohydrates from your diet and their replacement by fat.

By removing sugar from your diet and replacing it with foods high in fat, you allow your body to run on the fuel it was designed to run on.

Today we consume so much sugar every day that it is estimated that each American eats over 50 kilograms of sugar a year. As shocking as this is, it is rising so fast each year that some nutritional scientists have joked that it will reach 100% of the average American's diet by 2050.

Control Your Blood Sugar

The main goal of the Decarb Diet is to teach you how to control your blood sugar.

By controlling your blood sugar, you can control your insulin levels and insulin is the hormone that is keeping you fat. As soon as you stop eating carbs, your blood sugar levels will fall and down your insulin levels will go.

Keeping your insulin levels low will give your pancreas (which makes insulin) a chance to recover from the exhaustion caused by years of high carbohydrate bombardment.

You can eat as much as you want but you have to limit carbs because carbs stimulate insulin and too much insulin makes you fat and sick.

Once you understand what causes your individual blood sugar levels to rise and fall, you will have the tools to control your insulin levels and stay healthy and lean.

WHY YOU HAVE TO BALANCE YOUR OMEGA'S

Our food supply contains a massive oversupply of omega-6 fatty acids. Omega-3 fatty acids, on the other hand are scarce. A normal ratio of these two fatty acids is about one to one (1:1). However most of us have ratios of ranging from ten to twenty omega-6's to one omega-3 (10:1 to 20:1) in our tissues.

Why Is Omega-3 So Important?

Our brains are built from omega-3's, which make up about 25% of the brain's tissue. Omega-3's also form a vital part of the membranes in our bodies and the lack of omega-3 in our diet causes our membranes to become loaded with omega-6's. This is really bad news for our health.

Omega-6 loaded membranes are stiff and slow. They then behave like partially blocked drains, allowing only a reduced fluid flow. Thus nutrients pass more slowly into cells and waste extraction is in turn hindered.

Many scientists today believe that overloaded omega-6 membranes are part of the root cause of the degenerative heart and nerve diseases that plague our civilisation.

Hydrogenated Oils

Omega-3's are flexible and agile. They are also fragile, making foods with high omega-3 levels incompatible with a long shelf life. Thus, in order to prevent spoilage, food manufacturers remove them from their products. One of the processes they use is to hydrogenate the fatty acids, resulting in the terms 'partially hydrogenated' or 'hydrogenated' on food labels. Try to avoid eating these kinds of foods.

Never forget that we need both omega-6 and omega-3 in our diet. It is only because we eat so much omega-6 that the balance of the two gets out of whack.

William Lands

I found the best description of the problem when watching a series of video lectures by Dr William Lands, the world's foremost authority on essential fatty acids.

In these lectures, Lands highlights how our diet affects the composition of our tissues.[6] He also explains how the imbalance between 6's and 3's in our food supply is damaging our health.

Competition of the Omegas

Omega-6 and omega-3 fatty acids compete for parking space in our cell membranes. If you have a higher level of omega-3's in your diet, this will translate to a higher level of omega-3's in your membranes. So you have to increase your consumption of 3's **and at the same time** reduce your consumption of 6's.

Following the decarb diet eating and lifestyle plan will limit your exposure to omega-6's but you will still need to supplement with omega-3's to reach a healthy ratio of 6's to 3's. This healthy ratio is called the omega balance.

To enhance your omega-3 levels, I recommend that you eat lots of fish and leafy greens. However, you will still need to take a daily supplement of omega-3's of between 1 and 2 grams to achieve omega balance.

READ MORE You can find a complete explanation about why it is so important for your health to aim for an omega balance in your body, in the section 'Achieving Omega Balance is Critical for Your Health', p. 103.

READ MORE The suggested dosage and specific type of supplement is explained in the section 'Recommended Supplements', p. 44.

WHY YOU DON'T HAVE TO EXERCISE – BUT YOU SHOULD ANYWAY

Weight **loss** has nothing to do with exercise.

Because of this, the Decarb Diet does not prescribe exercise to lose weight. However, regular exercise will help keep off the weight you have lost.

Exercise also has many other proven health benefits. Exercising regularly helps you to stay lean by lowering your blood sugar levels and increasing the insulin sensitivity of your muscles.

Thus, I suggest that some exercise should always be part of your lifestyle. Moving your body is also important. For example, sitting for long periods is bad for you. Simply standing up once every twenty minutes can make a profound difference to your health and to your body's ability to burn fat.

Exercise has nothing to do with weight loss, but it has everything to do with wellness and staying lean.

READ MORE See the sections 'Exercise to Lose Weight? Sorry it is Not Going to Work!' p. 110 and 'The Hidden Dangers of Sitting', p. 113.

ASSESS YOURSELF

Answer these questions quickly:

- *Do you have a family history of diabetes or heart disease?*
- *Are you overweight or do you have a tendency to put on weight?*
- *Do you have tummy fat?*
- *Do you have sugar cravings?*
- *Do you find losing weight difficult?*
- *Has your doctor ever told you that your blood sugar is a little high?*
- *Are you doing less than 30 minutes of exercise twice a week?*
- *Do you have high blood pressure?*

Answered yes to one or more of these questions?

Then you can be pretty sure that you either have diabetic tendencies (with out-of-control blood sugar levels) or there is a good chance that you will eventually develop Type II diabetes.

Obesity is the leading cause of preventable death in the USA and most of the world.

Obesity takes years out of your life and life out of your years.

Take steps to heal yourself.

Follow the Decarb Program.

Act now!

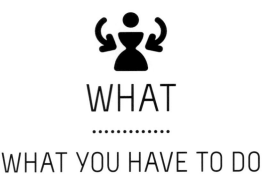

WHAT

WHAT YOU HAVE TO DO

This section contains the practical stuff you need to do to decarb and start your weight loss program. The program has three phases: Preparation, Strike and Stabilisation.

Preparation
During this phase you will measure your baselines, set your goals, prepare your kitchen and brush up on your decarb shopping skills.

Strike
Strike allows you to approach your goal weight by modifying your diet to exclude as many carbohydrates as possible. This phase normally takes eight weeks but can be longer if your weight loss is slower. Besides producing weight loss, Strike aims to teach you about your personal level of carbohydrate resistance.

Once you understand how your body handles carbs and how carbohydrate resistant you really are, you can use this knowledge to manage your eating patterns for the rest of your life.

Stabilisation
Stabilisation is about maintaining your weight with a low carb and high fat diet. It allows you to find out how many and what types of carbs you can gradually put back into your diet.

Recommended Supplements

A few supplements are recommended as part of this diet. Of these the omega-3 fish oil supplement is by far the most important.

- Omega-3 fish oil (EPA & DHA) – 1 to 2 grams a day
- Coenzyme Q10 – 100 to 200 mg a day
- Magnesium – 200 to 400 mg per day of elemental magnesium
- Vitamin D – 1,000 to 2,000 IU a day

PREPARATION

During the Preparation phase, you will perform a number of steps that lay the groundwork necessary to give you the best chance of succeeding with the Decarb Diet.

I expect you to go through these steps properly and in a determined manner, since the act of preparation will strengthen your resolve and reduce your chances of failure. The steps are:

1. Measure your personal baseline numbers (values)

2. Set your goals

3. Prepare your kitchen

4. Learn how to read labels

5. Study the Shopping Survival guide and then go decarb shopping

6. Prepare yourself for when you eat out

7. Buy the supplements if you opt to use them

8. Study carefully how to avoid stress

9. Commit to a starting date!

WHAT

MEASURE AND RECORD YOUR BASELINES

We will use these values as our guidelines as we progress through to the Strike phase.

Please measure yourself and enter the information in the spaces below. (You can also enter these values online at DecarbDiet.com, where the system will evaluate your numbers and make some recommendations for you.)

Current weight: _____ (kg)

Height: _____ (m) _____ (cm)

Waist: _____ (cm) (measured 1 cm above your belly button)

Waist height ratio: _____ (Divide your waist measurement by your height – this is an important measure of your body fat distribution)

Now calculate your Body Mass Index. This estimates body fat and is calculated as weight divided by height squared = mass (kg) / height (in metres)^2.

BMI: _____

Check and see where your BMI falls in the chart on the next page.

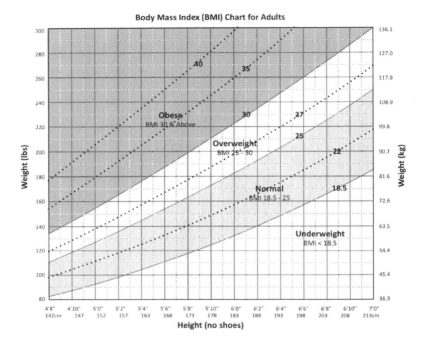

BMI Chart created by Vertex42.com. Used with permission.

Medical Tests

There are also two basic medical tests you should have done before you start the program, namely your fasting glucose (blood sugar) level and your blood pressure. These tests can be done at your local pharmacy (or by your doctor if you prefer).

Fasting Glucose Level

Simply wake up and go to your local pharmacy to get your glucose (blood sugar) tested before eating or drinking anything. Record your level here:

Fasting Glucose: _____

Blood Pressure
While you are having your blood sugar tested get your blood pressure done as well.

Blood Pressure Systolic: _____

Diastolic: _____

Optional Tests
These tests need to be done or ordered by your doctor.

Uric Acid: _____

HBA1c: _____ %

Blood Lipid Screening:

Total Serum Cholesterol: _____mmol/l

LDL ('bad') Cholesterol: _____mmol/l

HDL ('good') Cholesterol: _____mmol/l

Serum Triglycerides: _____mmol/l

If you are worried about your blood cholesterol levels, then it is a good idea to have a fasting lipogram ('cholesterol test') done before you start the diet. Then you can ask your doctor to redo the test after three to six months. In general most of my patients show improvements in this test after three months.

I suggest that you also have an HBA1c test before you start Decarb. Then have another at three to six months. The HBA1c test is good indication of your average blood sugar levels over the preceding eight weeks. A level of over 6.5 is a signal that you are pre-diabetic. Your levels will definitely come down as you progress through the program.

THE DECARB DIET: GUIDE TO A LOW CARB LIFESTYLE

SET YOUR PERSONAL GOALS

Target weight: _____

Goal 1: _____

Goal 2: _____

Goal 3: _____

Start date:

I will start my diet on the date below after I have made the necessary preparations.

Date: _____

Signed: _____

WHAT

PREPARE YOUR KITCHEN

One of the most important preparation steps is to make sure that your home is 'Carb Safe'. You do this by ridding your house of any foods, drinks or snacks that may trip you up in the early weeks of your decarb campaign.

Go through your kitchen, pantry, sweets cupboard and any other place where you stash snacks and remove anything that may threaten your resolve.

This step acts both as insurance and as a symbol of commitment to your diet goals. You may need to guard against that occasional mood or hormone change that will cause you to stray if the timing is right. If you happen to get home feeling miserable after a bad day – do you really need that chocolate bar, packet of sweets or tasty bread loaf to be staring you in the face? It would be so much better if you had prepared for this, by having the right food and snacks on hand to help you reach your goals.

In order to rid your kitchen of foods that will tempt you and sabotage your efforts, go through the checklist below and get rid of all the food items listed.

What to Remove

- Cold drinks (sodas) of any kind **including diet drinks**
- Fruit juice of any kind
- Flour of any kind – including whole wheat, buckwheat and other kinds of wheat
- Potatoes of any kind (yes, that includes sweet potatoes)
- Rice of any kind or colour
- Sugar of any type – including molasses, brown sugar, castor sugar, icing sugar, etc.
- Honey and syrups
- Artificial sweeteners – Xylitol and all similar types ending in '... ol' as well as any other sweeteners

- All food labeled 'lite' or 'diet' – like lite yoghurt or yoghurt with fruit
- All fruit except for the berry family
- All sweets and chocolates including chewing gum
- Any foods with the word hydrogenated in the label
- All vegetable oils

Finally, check all the food in your kitchen that comes in any kind of packaging – boxes, tins, etc. If it comes packaged, it probably needs to go, so read the ingredients list carefully.

- If you see sugar, carbohydrate, glycaemic carbs or the word 'hydrogenated' in the contents, then throw the stuff out.
- If you see the word fructose – throw.
- If you see words like corn syrup – throw. In South Africa this is usually referred to as HFCS (high fructose corn syrup).

Suggestion for Those Who Share Their Kitchen with Non-Dieters

Make a special place for 'forbidden foods' and keep them there. Make sure that the non-dieters understand why these foods are being kept in a separate place. Try to get their co-operation.

The forbidden food locker should be in a cupboard or a place that is discretely out of sight and can be kept closed. The aim is to make it difficult for you to take food from the locker. This will serve to deter you in those momentary lapses of resolve.

LEARN TO READ LABELS

In order to succeed as a decarber, you need to be constantly aware of the danger of unknowingly eating carbs. The worst possible case is to find out that an item that you are eating regularly has more carbohydrates than you realised. This item would be quietly sabotaging your efforts, spiking your insulin each time you ate it and silently stalling your fat-burning drive.

Net Carbs (Digestible Carbs or Glycaemic Carbs)

Make sure that you understand what Net Carbs are! This term refers to the digestible portion of carbohydrate in your serving and means the same thing as Digestible or Glycaemic Carbs.[7]

The carbs in a food source are often made up of a digestible portion and fibre, which is not digestible. The number given for total carbohydrates includes both of these. In order to calculate the actual carbs that will affect your blood sugar you need to know the Net Carb value.[8] Sometimes the food label will tell you, but not always.

For example, a packet of rice lists 77 grams of carbohydrates in a 100 gram portion, and less than half a gram of sugar.

Like this:

TYPICAL NUTRITIONAL INFORMATION		Sounds like something you can eat because it is low in sugar (0.4 grams)? Not! Look again at the label. It lists Glycaemic Carbohydrate at 77 grams. This is the business end of the stuff. Eat it and it will raise your blood sugar higher than the price of petrol.
Average values	per 100 g (uncooked)	
Energy	1500 kJ	
Protein	8,6 g	
Glycaemic carbohydrate of which total sugar	77 g 0,0 g	
Total fat	0,8 g	

Even a packet of wild brown rice contains a scant 1 or 2 grams of fibre. So despite all the 'healthy for you' marketing blurb on the packet, this rice packs a potent carb punch that will make you fat in no time.

Sugar Alcohols

These are often added to low carb or 'lite' products to reduce the sugar content and the glycaemic index. They mostly end in '... ol' – like xylitol, sorbitol etc.

They are not a free meal and do count as carbs even though they will not raise your blood sugar sharply and thus stimulate insulin release. In general, they can be added in to your Net Carbs calculation at **half** their listed carb value.

More on Reading Nutrition Information Labels

On the pages that follow I present a series of product nutrition information labels and explain how to read them. I suggest that you go through the examples and learn to spot the important (dangerous) ingredients.

You are most interested in:

- Glycemic carbs (sugars) – the stuff we are trying to avoid
- Portion size

Example: Full Fat Cream
I recommend cream as a milk substitute. It has less carbs than milk, tastes better and has the major benefit of making you feel full a whole lot quicker than milk does. (If you have to have milk, make sure it is full cream and not a low fat variety that has substituted milk sugar for the wholesome fat.)

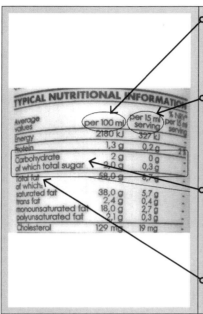

○ The 100 ml column here is useless until you know the actual container size, in this case 250 ml.

○ The serving size of 15 ml is an average portion size and you can usually estimate your carb load from values in this column.

○ These are the numbers that we are most interested in! We want to know total carbohydrates that are glycaemic (i.e. will cause insulin to rise).

○ Believe it or not, this cream is good stuff to eat!

Example: Balsamic Vinegar

Balsamic vinegar is a common ingredient in salads and is viewed as a healthy choice. It may be, but be cautious how much of it you pour onto your salad. A quick read of the label below should alarm you enough to know that this particular brand needs to be applied sparingly. (Since balsamic vinegar is made by double fermenting various fruits, the carb count will vary widely between brands; make sure you select a low carb variety.)

This balsamic vinegar has a lot of carbs! A tablespoon (15 ml) will have almost 6 grams of carbs. Be careful to use only a small amount; a big splash of this stuff could ruin your whole day.

Example: Breakfast Cereal

Remember that it is the glycaemic carbs that affect your blood sugar levels. There is no prize for figuring out that this stuff will make you fat.

TYPICAL NUTRITIONAL INFORMATION		
Average Values	per 100 g	per 45 g serving
Energy	1518 kJ	683 kJ
Protein	12,4 g	5,6 g
Glycaemic carbohydrate	58 g	26 g
of which total sugar	10,6 g	4,8 g
Total fat	6,5 g	2,9 g
of which:		

This breakfast cereal is hardly the breakfast of champions! One serving has 26 grams of carbs.

You would consume your entire day's allocation of carbs in one bowl!

Example: Sugar, the King of Carbs

Sugar, as you will have realised by now, is the star of the show in terms of packing on weight and damaging your health.

> *'... if only a small fraction of what is already known about the effects of sugar were to be revealed in relation to any other material used as a food additive, that material would promptly be banned.'* [9]
>
> John Yudkin, *Pure White and Deadly*

Note the conversion at the bottom of the image below from a sugar packet. One teaspoon of sugar equals 4-5 grams of carbs.

NUTRITIONAL INFORMATION		
Typical Values	per 100 g** as packed	per 4 g serving (as packed)
Energy	1698 kJ	68 kJ
Protein	0 g	0 g
Glycaemic Carbohydrate	100 g	(4 g)
of which		
total sugar	100 g	4 g
Total Fat	0 g	0 g
of which		
saturated fat	0 g	0 g
trans fat	0 g	0 g
monounsaturated fat	0 g	0 g
polyunsaturated fat	0 g	0 g
Dietary Fibre	0 g	0 g

Nice glycaemic load here!

As a rule of thumb 1 teaspoon of sugar equals almost 5 grams of carbs. Just imagine 7 teaspoons of this stuff in your Coke or 9 of them in your 'healthy' fruit juice.

WHAT

Example: Maize (Corn/Mealie Meal)

Maize is a cereal grain that is part of the staple diet of many people throughout the world, including the majority of South Africans.

It is America's largest crop and corn is grown on over 400,000 American farms.[10] Sweetcorn is a genetic variant. Corn is high in carbs and has very little fibre. Somewhere around 6% of America's corn crop is converted to High Fructose Corn Syrup and appears in many foodstuffs.

Corn and High Fructose Corn Syrup should be avoided.

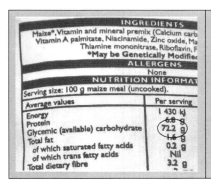

Maize (Mielie Meal)

Almost pure starch with little fibre, even though it is low in sugar. A bowl of this stuff should give your pancreas, which makes insulin, something to think about! Eat at your own risk.

Example: Wholewheat Pasta

Don't eat pasta – here's why!

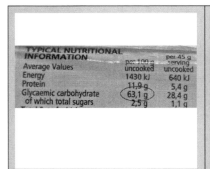

Pasta

Most pasta is about 70% pure carbs. Highly active and easy to digest, it quickly spikes blood sugar and since it is usually eaten in big bowlfuls it is a danger to be avoided.

THE DECARB DIET: GUIDE TO A LOW CARB LIFESTYLE

SUPERMARKET SURVIVAL

This section has some advice on how to survive in your supermarket and some tips on how to make the correct choices while doing your Decarb shopping.

You can make or break your Decarb efforts with the goods you choose to load into your trolley. Make no mistake, the aisles of a supermarket are a minefield for us decarbers.

An unbreakable rule is: **Avoid any products you see advertised on TV.**

The more advertising a product gets, either in-store or in other media, the more sure you can be that it is not something you want to put in your body. The better it is advertised, the poorer the quality of food you will get.

Another important rule is: **Avoid products that stress how healthy they are and ones that proudly sport 'medically proven' 'good for you' badges.**

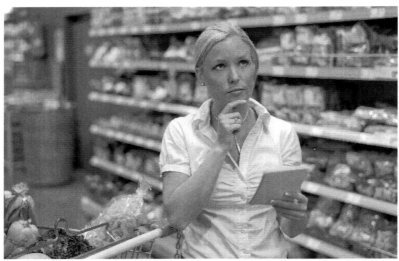

© Gina Sanders - Fotolia.com

The most important tool you need is your ability to read labels. So make sure that you have understood the principles of decoding food labels in the previous section.

Breakfast is a critical meal that can so easily become sugar laden and ruin your day. Do not buy any cereals – so you can skip the cereal aisle in the supermarket. Head for the dairy section and find some high fat natural, unsweetened yogurt. Look for some cheese – any kind will do except the low fat varieties.

Oils – Avoid all vegetable oils. Rather pick olive oil (extra virgin, which is the least refined) or coconut oil for cooking. A good tip for oils is to go for the darker varieties because, in general, the lighter coloured the oil is, the more it has been processed.

Fats – Butter is good. The program recommends that you increase your use of butter, so always keep a good stock of it. Never use margarine (except for polishing your car tyres). Avoid any product that lists hydrogenated fats and trans-fats among the ingredients.

Sauces – Avoid most of these. Tomato sauce is a big suspect in this area; it is high in sugar and salt and it is best to do without it altogether. Most tomato sauce contains corn starch, high fructose corn syrup, or similar ingredients. Check the labels of all salad dressings and other sauces carefully before you fling them into your trolley. Look carefully for sugar content before you buy. Rather choose sauces made of more natural products, which do not contain sugar or carbs.

Sweets – There is unfortunately very little you can buy in the sweet aisle. However 85% dark chocolate makes for a good treat. The Lindt variety has just over 1 gram of carbs per square.

Nuts – Buy good unprocessed, unsalted nuts. They make excellent snacks and can be added to meals as fillers and to salads.

READ MORE Details of which nuts to choose can be found in the 'Allowed Foods' section in Strike, p. 60.

Fruit – Avoid fruit because most fruit today is enhanced to carry excessive amounts of sugar and fructose and will quickly make you fat. A 'good fruit' is avocados: buy lots of these, and eat them as snacks or use as fillers for various dishes. Berries are also a good choice and an occasional apple is also OK. (Reminder: Fruit has a lot of fructose in it. Fructose is the single most important sugar for you to avoid. It is at the centre of what is making us fat and it lights the fire that results in many chronic and deadly diseases.)

Dried Fruit – Don't eat any dried fruit unless you are forced to do so at gunpoint. Most dried fruit is at least 50% sugar.

Fresh Produce – Leafy vegetables (greens) are all good. So are other vegetables except for the few that are high in carbs, which include potato, sweet potato, beans, squash and lentils.

Carrots are medium to low carb and can be eaten in moderate quantities. A cup of chopped carrots will have about 7 grams of glycaemic carbs. If you are trying to keep your daily carbs below 50 grams, then a cup of carrots will be more than 10% of your entire daily allotment.

Pumpkin is similar to carrot and has medium to low carbs – 6 grams a cup.

READ MORE See the Vegetable Carbs List in the Toolkit, p. 137.

Meat and Chicken – Where possible look for free range varieties. Avoid low-cost protein, which inevitably has antibiotics and hormones in it.

Fish – Sardines, salmon and herring are good sources of omega-3. Shrimp and scallops are good to eat and are low in toxins and mercury.

WHAT

SURVIVING EATING OUT

Sometimes you have to eat out. It may be dinner at a friend, a company lunch, or even when you are out with your family. There is no reason why you should stray from your low carb ways in these situations. Be strong and don't waiver too much or else you will be sorry the next day. Above all remember that no sugar or refined carbs are to pass your lips!

Eating Out Etiquette

A tip on good manners when eating out: simply pass when your host offers you carbs or other verboten concoctions. Try not to take this as an opportunity to launch into a low-carb evangelism lecture. Don't bring attention to yourself by announcing that you are a 'special eater' or that you have special eating requirements. This either inflames the 'eat anything and die happy' bigots or else raises the mother hen instinct in the bleeding hearts (to mix metaphors), who will go out of their way to help and eventually leave you no choice but to eat something totally inappropriate that they have dredged up for you in their effort to please.

Be resourceful and stealthy. For instance, if they are serving hamburgers and chips, simply discard the bun and the chips and eat the burger patty. Look for the cheese and cream that others will discard faster than nuclear waste, and load your plate.

Obviously you can always fall back on green salads and veggies. Just don't give in and eat the bread, the chips or the pasta.

Try not to eat out too often; it makes it much harder to control what you eat.

Eating out or ordering takeaways may be convenient, but if you're not careful, it can sabotage your weight management efforts. People who eat out tend to consume an average 500 more calories per meal than they would if they ate a similar meal at home. Meals eaten out translate into increased consumption of bad fats and higher carb intakes.

THE DECARB DIET: GUIDE TO A LOW CARB LIFESTYLE

RECOMMENDED SUPPLEMENTS

The four supplements below are recommended as part of the Decarb program. None of these supplements is an absolute requirement and you can lose weight without them but taking them will improve your health and will more than likely aid your weight loss and health efforts.

If you find your weight plateauing and you get stuck at a point where you seem to be getting no lighter, even though you are carefully watching your carb intake, then these supplements may be exactly what you need to break the deadlock.

- Omega-3 fish oil (EPA & DHA) – 1 to 2 grams a day
- Coenzyme Q10 – 100 to 200 mg a day
- Magnesium – 200 to 400 mg per day of elemental magnesium
- Vitamin D – 1,000 to 2,000 IU a day

If you decide to use supplements, you need to buy the right ones. What follows explains what to look for.

Omega-3 Fish Oil

At least 1 gram of EPA and DHA (combined) daily is recommended.

Take this fish oil supplement in order to help maintain a balance between the omega-6's and omega-3's in the tissues of your body.

READ MORE Please read more about this in the section 'Achieving Omega Balance is Critical for Your Health', p.103.

There is a lot of low quality fish oil available out there. It is usually not difficult to determine that a supplement is of low quality. If it is low priced it is probably best avoided. Low quality fish oil may contain mercury and other contaminants, so beware.

Good quality fish oil has the following attributes:

- It says that it is 'pharmaceutical-grade'
- It says that it is 'molecularly distilled'

NB: Make sure that the EPA and DHA quantities in the capsule or tablet that you select add up to about 1 gram. Cheaper varieties often have reduced levels of these two vital ingredients.

For example – the contents of a single 1,000 mg capsule are listed as:

- Concentrated Salmon Oil 1,000 mg
- EPA – 198 mg
- DHA – 132 mg

With this supplement your total omega-3 per capsule would be 330 mg (198 plus 132), so you would need to take three of these a day to get your recommended 1 gram (1,000 mg) a day.

Also remember to increase your intake of fish, especially salmon, sardines and other cold water fish, as part of your omega-3 intake.

Omega-3 Benefits

There is no doubt that omega-3 fish oil is good for your heart. As early as 1999 a study of over 11,000 patients who had suffered heart attacks, found that they were protected by a 1 gram daily dose of omega-3's. Patients on these supplements benefitted with an up to 45% reduction in sudden death, most likely caused by the anti-arrhythmic effects of the omega-3's.[11]

In summary, the benefits of omega-3 supplementation are:

- Decreases inflammation – general anti-inflammatory effects (mainly as a result of reducing the dominance of omega-6 fatty acids in cell membranes)
- Lowers blood pressure
- Reduces aggregation of platelets (reduces blood clot potential in your blood stream)

- Lowers you changes on heart arrhythmias
- Supports nerve and brain functions

Important Note: Flax Seed Oil

Try and use flax seed oil daily in addition to your fish oil capsules. It has high levels of ALA (alpha-linoleic acid) as well as moderate DHA and EPA levels. **The best way to do this is to make a habit of adding a tablespoon of flax seed oil to your salad.**

Flax seed oil can be used as a fish oil substitute. Note however that it has lower concentrations of EPA and DHA and thus needs to be taken in bigger doses. A tablespoon of flax seed oil has about 700 mg of EPA and DHA. This means that a single fish oil capsule would have to be replaced with at least four or more flax seed oil capsules of a similar size. Always keep your opened flax seed oil bottle in the fridge.

Flax meal can also be used; it is a good source of omega-3's as well as being high in fibre.

Coenzyme Q10

100 mg daily or twice daily is recommended.

Coenzyme Q10 (Co-Q10) helps your body energy systems to work efficiently. (It works on ATP, which is the body's energy molecule.)

Co-Q10 is closely related to the energy production systems of the body and although it can be found everywhere in the body, the highest concentration of Co-Q10 is found in the heart. One heart specialist claims that he found that up to 75% of his heart patients were deficient in Co-Q10.

The other benefits of Co-Q10 are:

- Anti-oxidant
- Skin repair and health
- May help to boost athletic performance
- Counteract the unwanted side-effects of statins

Statins reduce the body's ability to make Co-Q10, by directly interfering with the mevalonate pathway. This is the same pathway that leads to the production of cholesterol. **It is vital for anyone taking statins to supplement with Co-Q10.**

Magnesium

Low magnesium levels are strongly associated with increased insulin resistance. Many people who suffer from insulin resistance have low magnesium levels. A 2002 study found that 65% of individuals 192 individuals in the trial who had Insulin Resistance Syndrome (Metabolic Syndrome) also had low magnesium levels.[12]

Predisposing Factors and Symptoms of Magnesium Deficiency
If you have any of the symptoms or habits listed below, you may have a magnesium deficiency. The more of these you have, the more likely it is that you are magnesium deficient.

- Drink a lot of coffee
- Are frequently irritable or have mood swings
- Are frequently anxious
- Exercise a lot
- Take laxatives
- Heart palpitations
- Muscle cramps

Magnesium supplementation assists with:

- Osteoporosis prevention
- Migraine relief
- Chronic fatigue
- Reducing insulin resistance

Vitamin D

An alarming number of people are deficient in vitamin D.

Researchers have consistently found that between 30% and 80% of the US population is deficient in vitamin D. A 2011 study of 4,495 adult participants found that 82% of the black people in the study were vitamin D deficient.[13]

The reason for this is that few foods naturally contain vitamin D and people are spending less time in the sun. The widespread use of sunscreen preparations also reduces the skin's ability to make vitamin D.

Dairy products and certain fatty fish contain vitamin D. In addition, many foods such as cereals and milks are fortified with vitamin D. Vitamin D is vital for bone health, calcium absorption, controlling cell growth and immune function. It is also involved in the secretion of insulin and reduced vitamin D levels have been associated with reduced insulin secretion in patients with type 2 diabetes.[14, 15]

The following symptoms may indicate a vitamin D deficiency:

- You get flu often
- You suffer from muscle weakness
- You have itchy and dry skin
- Your fasting blood sugar levels are elevated
- You have gum disease or suffer from bleeding and sore gums

WHAT

STRESS

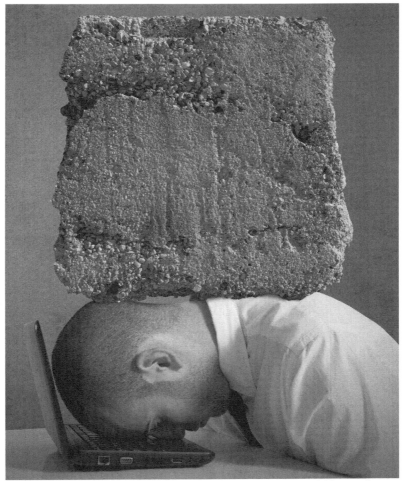

© Olena Pantiukh - Fotolia.com

Stress is an inescapable part of our everyday lives. You can speed up your weight loss efforts (or get over a weight loss plateau) by reducing your stress levels.

In our primal past, stress normally came in a sudden life-or-death moment, requiring immediate action. This is the kind of stress you would feel if an intruder suddenly appeared next to your bed in the night.

Acute stress like this seldom happens in real life. We suffer from a different kind of stress.

Chronic Stress

Most of us co-exist with chronic stress levels, something that we feel as an unrelenting background pressure, a state that we come to regard as 'normal'.

Living with chronic stress is more than an unpleasant feeling; it has physical effects and health risks. Chronic stress is a health hazard which can harm both your heart and your immune system. It also contributes to the progression of many diseases.

Hans Selye, who coined the word 'stressor', was the first to define stress in a biological context. He said that stress '... in addition to being itself, was also the cause of itself, and the result of itself'.[16]

Stressors

A stressor is a source of stress. Most stressors are mental, like the feeling of loss of control. Stressors can also be physical, for example having to work in an uncomfortable environment or having to deal with a physical problem such as a headache or flu. Other examples of stressors are traffic jams, queues, money problems and problems at work, as well as family issues and so many others.

We cannot avoid stressors in our lives; we need to modify how we react to stress.

Stress Hormones

Cortisol is the main stress hormone and high stress levels cause high cortisol levels. Cortisol inhibits the effects of other hormones such as growth hormones and sex hormones and reduces the body's ability to lose weight.

Some side-effects of chronic stress are:

- Poor blood sugar control
- Lower bone density and less muscle mass
- Higher deposits of abdominal fat
- Lower immunity to colds, flu and infections

Reducing Stress

First and foremost – recognise the big stressors in your life! Then take meaningful steps to reduce or adapt to them.

Some general measures:

- **Having good relationships with your family and friends is vital for your health.**
- Sleep more – less than 8 hours of sleep a night raises cortisol levels.
- Take a nap if you are feeling stressed.
- Watch your caffeine intake – especially at night. Consider a caffeine curfew and stop drinking caffeine-containing beverages like coffee after sundown.
- Plan more! Spend more time planning your days. Time taken planning daily activities is well spent. Good planning gives you a sense of control that greatly reduces stress.
- Laugh more and spend time with people who make you laugh.
- Exercise more. Exercise is a great way to reduce stress. You don't have to exercise for hours or push hard. A low-intensity twenty minute walk, jog or cycle will do wonders for your stress levels at the same time as being good for your heart.
- Have a massage – a good massage will lower the levels of all your stress hormones.

Exercise: List Your Stressors

Do you want to really reduce some of the stress in your life?

It is not hard to do. Take twenty minutes and sit down in a quiet place and compile a list of the top ten things that stress you most.

Once you have the list in front of you, go through it carefully and see if you can think of ways to reduce or remove any of the items on the list.

Check carefully for anything on the list that can be **handled differently** to the way you are currently dealing with it. Making a change in the way you respond to a stressor may make a massive difference to your life.

Also look at ways that better planning can be used to reduce the levels of stress or even remove items from your list.

STRIKE

Now the real work begins.

From today you will:

- Start your new carb-free diet
- Take your supplements if used
- Take regular measurements
- Stick to your chosen exercise routine
- Keep a journal

A Strike phase normally lasts eight weeks, and can be longer. Some people need only one Strike phase to reach their goal weights; others may need more.

You need to continue in Strike until you reach within 10% of your goal weight.

Aim of the Strike Phase

Your aim is to eat as few carbs as possible during the initial 8 weeks of the diet. Always aim at 25 grams per day but know that you have some leeway and you will be OK as long as you don't go over 50 grams on any given day.

Your goal is to remove carbs and replace them with fat and protein. The carbs you remove will be replaced by high fat, protein-based foods, with some vegetables. Your current daily diet probably contains between 250 to 300 grams of carbs. It is not difficult to remove the first few hundred grams of carbs. Just stop eating all the foods listed in the Forbidden Foods section below. By now you have a good idea of what these foods are.

Sugar Cravings

You may have to deal with sugar cravings during the initial weeks of Strike. This is normal. In some ways it will be similar to giving up smoking or alcohol.

The best way to deal with sugar cravings is to eat some fatty food, preferably with some protein. This will quickly make you feel full and will normally quench the craving. Giving in and having a quick bite or two of something sweet should be avoided at all costs.

Remember sugar cravings are part of a carbohydrate addiction and you cannot be feeding the craving with sugar! Imagine if alcoholics were advised to have a little drink each time they felt the need.

Believe it or not, eventually you will lose your taste for sweet things, usually after a month or two. Once you get to that stage you will be amazed to find that you can't eat the sweet stuff anymore, or at least not in the same quantities as you used to.

Sweeteners

I am often asked if sweeteners are allowed. The answer is a qualified yes. There is no dietary reason why you should not replace the sugar in your drinks with a sweetener. This will greatly reduce the insulin rise that the sugar would produce.

However, I don't like sweeteners! If you absolutely have to use them then do so, rather than using sugar. But be aware that most of the popular sweeteners available today, including aspartame and sucralose, are artificially created compounds that you have no business drinking on a regular basis. A number of sources go so far as to call them poisons. If you have any doubts then Google the chemical name of your favourite sweetener.

If your ultimate goal is to reduce the sugars in your diet, you will never get achieve that if you keep stimulating your sweet tooth. Thus I strongly recommend that you do not use sugar replacements in your drinks because it perpetuates your sugar dependency.

Be as Lean as You Can Be

You can be as lean as you want to be; you just have to remove enough carbs from your diet.

You need never be hungry during Strike.

Don't overeat. Listen to your body and eat only when you are hungry.

Eat slowly and eat only as much of the allowed foods as you need to.

You don't need carbs to survive! Humankind managed fine for two million years without carbs – so can you.

FORBIDDEN FOODS

Below is a list of forbidden foods.

Some of these will always be forbidden – such as sugar, honey, fructose, fizzy drinks, fruit juice, margarines, vegetable oils and cereals. Others, like fruit, full cream milk and rice, can be added back in the Stabilisation Phase, once you are within 10% of your target weight.

© Olena Pantiukh - Fotolia.com

These foods are all forbidden during the Strike phase:

- Sugar (white, brown or any colour at all)
- Honey, syrup or any substitute such as (high fructose) corn syrup
- Bread of any kind whatsoever, including, muffins, rolls, bagels
- Milk
- Fruit of any kind except berries
- Fruit juices of any kind
- Fructose in any form
- Low fat, sweetened or fruit yoghurt
- Diet drinks, fizzy or sweetened drinks: Coke, Pepsi and all others

WHAT

- Beer, wine, fizzy alcoholic drinks, cocktails
- Starches of any kind (potatoes, rice, couscous, noodles, quinoa)
- Pasta of any kind, including wholewheat pasta
- Any grains – including whole grains, corn and sweetcorn
- Potato chips (crisps) of any kind
- Any cereals – corn flakes, rice crispies, oats, oat bran, etc.
- Margarines, canola oils and most vegetable oils
- Beans and legumes
- Carrots
- Peas
- Cashew nuts and peanuts (**Cashew nuts** *are little packets of carbs.* **And never eat peanuts!** *They are packed with carbs and contain massive quantities of omega-6's.*)
- Salad dressings that have sugar in them

WHAT ELSE TO WATCH OUT FOR

The list of 'forbidden items' can never be complete without your help. Sugar and refined carbs infest our food supply so you will have to be eternally vigilant.

Remember that any carbs that slip through your guard will raise your blood sugar and create a temporary setback. These unwanted carbs will raise your insulin levels and slow down fat breakdown.

Be savvy and be alert. If you start eating anything that tastes sweet – just stop, it is better to be safe than sorry.

Look out for hidden sugars; many cooked items are made with sugar and other carb sweeteners, which 'they' forget to tell you about.

Some Places You Might Find Hidden Danger

- Sauces
- Salad dressings
- Cooked vegetables
- Balsamic vinegar – certain varieties can pack a big carb punch
- Fructose used as sweetener
- Honey hidden in a 'no-sugar' treat

I cannot stress how deadly fructose is for you. A glass of water with fructose (or sugar, which is half fructose) is liquid fat in a glass. Fructose goes straight to your liver and is converted into triglycerides which are then stored directly as fat, either in your liver or else transported to the body's fat stores.

Always Read the Labels

Be wary; there are carbs everywhere and you will need to be a detective to avoid the hidden carbs that are thrown at you.

A study by the University of Carolina bought 85,451 uniquely formulated (branded) items from US supermarkets between

2005 and 2009 and then tested each of these items for sugar. An astounding 75% of these contained **added** sugar, which in many cases was not discernible from the Nutrition Facts labelling.[17]

Examine food labels for key words such as carbohydrates, glycaemic sugars, glycaemic 'anything', sugars and starch. Read and re-read the section on Learn How to Read Labels.

Avoid eating any food that lists 5 grams or more of carbohydrates on the ingredients label.

You are not alone. If you need advice or help with any item please mail support@Decarbdiet.com and we will do our best to assist you.

Sugar Has Many Names

Do not be fooled by the names some manufacturers give the sugar in their products. Here is a list of some of the trade names that sugar and carbs hide behind:

Sucrose, fructose, maltose, lactose, honey, agave syrup, brown-rice syrup, molasses, corn sweetener, corn syrup, cane juice, etc.

READ MORE Sugar: Sweet Suicide, p.86

ALLOWED FOODS

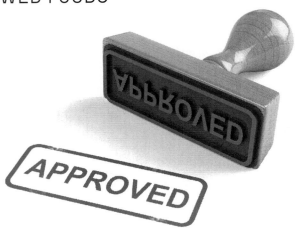

Protein
Eat as much as you need to of:

- Meat – any kind of unprocessed meat is allowed but **grass fed** is preferred
- Poultry – chicken, turkey and duck – free range is **always** preferred!
- Fish – any seafood

(Try to reduce your consumption of processed meats such as sausages, hot dogs, ham and bacon. Ensure that the sausages you eat do not contain carbs by reading the labels carefully.)

Remember: Aim for high fat – do not avoid fatty portions!

Vegetables
- Green salads are allowed and encouraged! Always eat lots of greens. But beware of the dressings you use as these often contain sugar
- Tomato, green vegetables
- Spinach/broccoli/celery

- Avocado (eat as much as you want)
- Mushrooms, peppers, chillies
- Onions

Dairy Products and Eggs
- Whole eggs with no restriction – fry in butter, coconut oil or ghee
- Cheese
- Full fat cream
- Full cream yoghurt
- Butter – use as much as you want, to cook with

Other
- Olive oil and flax seed oil – use freely
- Lard/coconut oil/ghee – use for frying in place of vegetable or canola oil.
- Nuts (listed here from the most desirable, lowest carb count, to the least desirable)
  - Macadamia (highest fat)
  - Pecans
  - Brazils
  - Hazels
  - Almonds
- Mayonnaise – full fat variety, but use sparingly, as mayonnaise is packed with omega-6's.

Drinks
Love water! Try hard to get used to drinking water. Because of our exposure to years of sweet drinks, we have forgotten our love of plain, pure cold water.

Try and rediscover your love of water. You really don't need to drink anything else to survive. However, you may drink tea and coffee, preferably without sweeteners (see below).

Alcohol

Spirits – vodka, whisky, gin and rum – are allowed in moderation. Never to be mixed with anything except water or ice.

Treats

- Biltong between meals
- Nuts and cheese slices
- 85% Lindt chocolate; it tastes like spray-painted cardboard, but provides comfort food (each piece has just over 1 gram of carbs)

Sweeteners

If you need to you can use small amounts of sweeteners. But try hard to limit your use of these because they keep your taste buds accustomed to sweet tastes, something we are trying hard to get un-used to.

Always remember that this is a high fat diet and you need to eat fat. It is not always easy to do this but if you do, your appetite will be naturally diminished and you will not be hungry for hours at a time.

Try to break the ingrained habit of always looking for low-fat foods.

- Don't choose lean cuts when buying meat.
- Eat the fatty bits when you eat protein.
- Eat the skin of the chicken.
- Don't pick the low-fat cheese or cottage cheese.
- Don't buy or eat low-fat anything.

Always choose high fat, to replace carbs. Eating fat quickly makes you feel full.

SOME EXAMPLES OF LOW CARB MEALS

Breakfast

- Eggs – fried, scrambled. Use lots of butter to fry the eggs
- Omelettes with cheese, meat or tomato
- Full cream yoghurt – you can mix more cream in with your yoghurt
- Meat – add bacon or other meat to your eggs

It is **vital** that you have a good fat source in your breakfast meal.

The fat content is the key. It is calorie dense and fills you up. Since your blood sugar levels do not go up like they do when you eat toast or cereals, you will not feel the classic mid-morning hunger pangs.

Lunch

Your best option is meat or another source of protein.

- Meat, fish or poultry
- Vegetables and greens
- Cheese slices or high fat cream cheese

If your protein source is lean you need to add some fat to the meal. Add full fat cream, an avocado, high fat salad dressing or cheese, as necessary.

Dinner

Same as lunch.

Snacks

- Fatty biltong always works well. A small amount will normally fill you up
- Cheese slices are good
- Coffee with lots of cream is also filling

THE DECARB DIET: GUIDE TO A LOW CARB LIFESTYLE

READ MORE Look at the Recipes in the Toolkit, p. 146, but remember that they may be more suitable for the Stabilisation phase, not the strict Strike phase.

RECORDING YOUR PROGRESS

Regular Weighing

I suggest that you weigh yourself once a week. This will warn you of gradual changes in your body weight and prevent one of those shocking moments when you try on something that used to fit perfectly and it dawns on you that you have "put on weight".

Weigh yourself at more or less the same time each week, so that your readings remain consistent. Record your results! Do not rely on memory. You can use the journal provided in the Toolkit, or the online version on the DecarbDiet.com website to enter your readings.

Measuring

Body measurements should be done monthly. These will help to highlight the changes that happen to your body as a result of your Decarb Lifestyle. Often weight levels may stay the same, while your body measurements will reveal how your shape has changed.

Keep a Journal

As well as recording your weight and body measurements, and the amount of exercise you take, it is very useful to record how you feel, what was easy, what was difficult, and so on. See the Journal section in Toolkit, p.167.

STABILISATION

The Stabilisation phase is also known as the Recarb phase. In this phase you replace some of the less bad carbs; you are not expected to live on a carb-free diet forever!

The earliest you can start Stabilisation is when you are within 10% of your goal weight and have maintained that weight for at least a month.

When you get here, well done! You have lived through the hard part of weaning yourself off the carbs and now you need to settle into a routine and lifestyle that will keep you lean for the rest of your life.

But be careful, this phase is dangerous.

Make no mistake, the initial few months of Stabilisation are the most dangerous time for you. You have achieved so much and it can all go down the drain so fast.

Do you really want to look back at your achievements a year from now only to find that you have slowly slipped back into your old carb habits and the lost weight has crept back?

It can happen so easily. When you Recarb you need to be cautious and resist the temptation to give yourself too much leeway with your choices.

Treat yourself like a reformed alcoholic and stay well away from the sweet stuff. Never forget that you were overweight and have all the necessary capabilities to become overweight again.

How it Works

During the Stabilisation phase carbs are slowly added to the diet and weight is monitored weekly.

Start by selecting one carb to add to the foods you are eating. Then over the next few weeks, watch to see if you stop losing weight or even gain weight again. This is a slow but necessary process.

Unfortunately there is no prescription that will work for everyone. Each of us has an individual response to carb loads, which changes as we age.

It goes without saying that the carbs you add will not be of the high glycaemic index (GI), heavily processed variety. If you have reached this phase you should have got the message by now that sugar is your enemy. So add 'good' carbs back carefully.

If you feel yourself getting hungry again – then consciously eat some more fat and protein. This will get your appetite under control again.

Stabilisation is a personal journey. Go slowly and be careful as you add back carbs. Try to add them back one at a time, and wait a while to ensure that you understand the effects. If you add items individually it will help you to discover which carb choices don't agree with you.

An important tool during this phase is your Blood Glucose tester. By monitoring your blood sugar levels on waking and every 2 hours you will get a really good idea of how the newly added carbs affect you.

Maintain Your Good Habits!

Just because you are in Stabilisation don't forget to maintain your journals:

- Weigh yourself once a week
- Record your measurements at least once a month

Be alert to changes in your body. Be warned if your clothes start feeling tight or if you suddenly feel a little thicker or more rounded somewhere.

If you feel that you have gained weight and your measurements show it, act quickly to stop the slide. You know how to fix it! Just take some more carbs out of your diet for a few weeks and you will soon be back to normal.

The key is to be vigilant and not to slip into complacency, buoyed by your past success. Also remember that your health will suffer and your energy levels will decline if you put weight back on.

PLATEAU BUSTING

There are two kinds of plateaus that may affect you. (You 'plateau' when you stop losing weight on a diet, usually despite still wanting to lose more and despite sticking to the diet.) One type of plateau typically happens early in the program; the other happens later.

Weight Loss Suddenly Stops

This is a common problem, which typically goes like this:

You start on Decarb and for the first few weeks you lose weight but then suddenly your weight loss drops off, leaving you with weight still to lose.

The most common cause of this problem is you have started to relax the control of your carb intake. Normally this happens after you have removed all the big carb baddies from your diet but there are some smaller sources of carbs left that are now sabotaging your efforts.

So if you are stuck in an in-diet plateau, my first suggestion is to go carefully over the food you eat regularly, meal by meal, and look for the hidden source of carbs.

Remember that we try for a carb intake of less than 25 grams during the Strike phase. Make sure that you really are within this limit. Now stay at or below 25 grams of carbs a day for another two weeks and watch to see if your weight loss restarts.

If after these additional two weeks, you are still stuck, then consider a temporary increase in the amount you exercise for a two or three week period. This should break you out of your plateau.

If you are **still** stuck, then consider trying Intermittent Fasting as discussed in the next section.

You can also mail support@decarbdiet.com for more personalised advice.

Stubborn Weight

For many of my patients, being on Decarb brings good results.

Their weight comes down and their health improves and all is good. They find a balance between avoiding carbs at all costs and an occasional transgression or treat, which still enables them to stabilise at an acceptable weight.

Unfortunately for some, that balance point is reached before those last few pounds are gone, leaving a small residue of fat around the midsection or elsewhere.

Sometimes we ask too much of our bodies. We need to accept that we can't all look like athletes on TV or movie stars on the beach. But if you feel that you need to get leaner, then you probably can; it is just going to take some hard work and dedication, which is exactly what some of the stars go through to look so good in the first place!

If you are in this position my first recommendation is to go back and check if there is any way you can tighten your carb control. Try to squeeze the last few carbs out of your diet for a few weeks and see if that helps. If you are **still** carrying extra weight then there are two additional methods that you can consider.

Increase your exercise intensity and volume

If you are exercise regularly, then you need to find creative ways to increase either your exercise volume or the intensity at which you exercise. If you are not on a regular exercise program – then now is the time to start!

- It is better to exercise twice a day for twenty minutes than to do a single forty minute session once a day. If you can, try and exercise twice a day, once or twice a week.
- In general morning exercise sessions are better than evening sessions.
- If you do mainly cardio exercise routines, consider adding a regular session of resistance training. Resistance training is really good for increasing muscle insulin sensitivity.

- Make one of your cardio sessions shorter but really hard.

If you are already doing regular resistance training, consider a 'primal' session once a week. By primal I mean a routine that emphasises maximal effort over a short duration. For example: pick five resistance exercises that engage large muscle mass (see the example below). Then after a good warm-up, do just a single set of each of these five exercises, between 6 and a maximum of 12 repetitions. The idea is to push as much weight as you possibly can in a single set. If can manage only six or fewer reps, this means the weight is too heavy for you. When you can exceed twelve reps on an exercise, you need to increase the weight at your next session. Keeping good notes will help. Your last rep really needs to be your last rep! Make an all-out effort with the five exercises, then go home. This kind of routine done once a week (only!) will produce a surge in hormones and a good rise in muscle insulin sensitivity.

Here is an example routine for a primal exercise session.

- Leg press
- Lat rows
- Pull-downs or pull-ups
- Bench press
- Triceps dips

Intermittent Fasting
Many diets incorporate the concept of IF (Intermittent Fasting). Some of these are wrongheaded efforts that propose a once or twice weekly fast, backed up by a food splurge for the rest of the week (the 5:2 Diet or the Fast Diet, for example). The problem with this kind of routine is that it does not address the real reasons the dieter has gained weight in the first place. It simply goes around the problem and leaves the dieter with ongoing health issues.

However, since these unhealthy diets do work in the short term, we can learn from them. I think that the reason they work is because of the value of the intermittent fast.

Think for a moment about our ancestors. They did not have the benefit of refrigeration to store food and as a result we can surmise that they awoke on many a morning with nothing to eat. This would then leave them with no choice but to go out and hunt or gather food. A consequence of occasional mornings or even days without food would be to embed a tolerance mechanism for intermittent fasting into our systems.

So my suggestion is that, if you are stuck in a plateau and are doing 'everything right', then a course of IF may help you to lose more weight.

My method of IF is simple and not painful at all. It involves an easy twelve to fifteen hour fast once or twice a week. It is easy because if you don't eat after dinner and sleep for eight hours, all you need to do is to skip breakfast; you can break your fast at lunchtime. Moreover you can drink water, tea and coffee as long as you use no milk, creamers or sugar.

Fear of Fasting
There is some fear attached to the concept of not eating. This is understandable, but give it a try and you will be amazed at how easy it is to go without eating. Somehow all the breakfast cereal ads in the world cannot overcome our built-in capability to get up and get going on an empty stomach.

Remember that the saying 'Breakfast is the most important meal of the day!' is just an advertising slogan designed to make us all eat more cereals.

WHAT

USING A GLUCOSE METER

Not everyone on the Decarb Diet will be motivated enough to measure their daily blood sugar levels with a blood glucose tester. It is important to take some blood sugar readings especially at the beginning to establish a baseline and to give yourself an idea of possible diabetic tendencies. The best way to do this is to go to a pharmacy and ask them to do the test for you. Start with an initial fasting level, taken soon after waking on an empty stomach.

If you find your initial casual test out of the normal range, then I strongly suggest that you get yourself a meter and start doing daily checks until you know exactly what is going on with your blood sugar. This is also an option for patients who get stuck.

READ MORE You can find information about normal 'Blood Sugar Levels' in the Toolkit, p. 144.

Testing Yourself

This is the shortest step and the hardest for most of us because we have to learn to prick ourselves with a needle. Not just once but up to three times a day. But don't worry, the tiny prick is almost painless and is necessary to draw a small drop of blood for the glucose meter you will use.

Daily testing will enable you to gain an understanding of how different meals and snacks affect your blood sugar levels. After all, the Decarb Diet is all about controlling your insulin levels by controlling how many carbs you feed into your system. The best way to achieve this is by monitoring actual blood sugar levels.

The use of a glucose meter may seem like overkill to you. It is not. If you are driving past a speed trap in your car, would you trust yourself to guess that you are travelling below the speed limit? In this case the cost of a wrong guess is just a fine, while if you get your blood sugar levels wrong it may cost you your health.

73

Initially you will need to measure blood sugar levels at least three times a day:

1. When you wake up (before eating or drinking)

2. Two hours after breakfast

3. Two hours after dinner

Obtaining a Glucose Meter

It is often possible to get a glucose testing unit free from your local pharmacy. These units are supplied 'for free' if you buy a pack of blood glucose test strips. This makes your outlay low, usually in the region of R200.

Most companies supply strips in packs of fifty, so your initial purchase should last you about 3 weeks. Generally after three weeks of monitoring you will have a good idea of your blood sugar levels in various situations. After that a pack of fifty test strips will last you a lot longer.

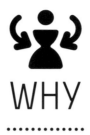

WHY

THE SCIENCE BEHIND THE DIET

Today the world is full of fat people and there is no consensus as to why. What we do know is that we are getting fatter and sicker. Obesity is everywhere, so much so that it almost seems normal for everyone around us to carry some extra weight.

This section deals with the theory and research behind the Decarb Diet. It is here for you to dip into as you feel the need to understand why the diet is structured as it is. Only by increasing our knowledge and understanding of what is going on around us can we hope to determine the best path to health and vibrant longevity.

On the next page is a picture of the fattest man in the world in the early 1900s. He was so unusual that people paid to see him at a circus freak show. Today we see people as fat as him on a daily basis.

THE DECARB DIET: GUIDE TO A LOW CARB LIFESTYLE

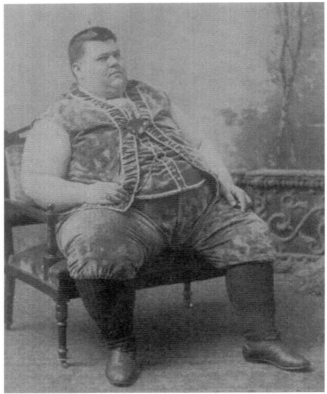

World's Fattest Man 1904

WHAT IS CARBOHYDRATE RESISTANCE?

Individuals with carbohydrate resistance (CR) are born with a genetically diminished capacity to handle carbohydrate in their diets. The capacity to handle carbohydrates varies from person to person. It also changes as an individual ages.

The concept was originally mooted as 'metabolic resistance' by Dr Robert Atkins.[18] 'His metabolic resistance to losing is so great that it has never been possible for him to lose when we tried adding any carbohydrate at all to his diet.'

Sugar in the Blood

Any carbohydrate that we eat gets broken down into glucose and other sugars, which are then absorbed into our bloodstream. (Glucose in the blood is called 'blood sugar'.) As the glucose begins to accumulate in your blood, your pancreas squirts insulin into the bloodstream to deal with the glucose. This is because glucose, although vital for life, is toxic and can only be handled in the blood in strictly limited quantities. On average, each person has no more than a single teaspoon of glucose in their blood. Very high glucose levels in your blood will quickly kill you, while constantly raised levels often lead to diabetes, heart disease and other life-diminishing problems.

Carb Resistant People Can Easily Deal With Fat

While carbohydrate resistant people have difficulty storing and metabolizing carbohydrate, they have no such difficulty dealing with fat.[19] Because of a difficulty in dealing with carbs, people with carbohydrate resistance (CR) need to produce more insulin to handle the carbs that they have eaten. This raised insulin level and the associated high blood sugar levels slowly get out of control.

The time it takes for this problem to become evident depends on your individual level of CR. The problem will initially be invisible. However, when your system starts to get overloaded you will put on weight, because your body, unable to deal with the glucose in your blood, will begin to store the glucose as fat in your fat cells. And slowly but surely you will get bigger.

As a rule of thumb, you can say that the more overweight you are, the more carbohydrate resistant you are. People with CR will store fat in their livers as well, which can lead to additional health issues.

Prevention of Obesity in Carbohydrate Resistant People

Prevention is easy. Simply avoid eating carbohydrates and increase the fat content of your diet and you will lose weight, which is exactly what the Decarb Diet proposes.

Initially all carbs are withheld from the diet, in order to produce the best possible weight loss. Then carbs are slowly fed back into the diet, until the patient begins to put on weight again. The point at which this occurs varies from person to person.

CR is for Life

Unfortunately your carbohydrate resistance does not go away if you lose weight. It is with you for life. The only sensible option that you have is to manage it by eating a low carb diet for the rest of your life and the best way to do that is by following the Decarb Lifestyle.

IS THERE SUCH A THING AS CARBOHYDRATE ADDICTION?

Yes there is.

Carbohydrate addiction is every bit as real as nicotine or recreational drug addiction.[20]

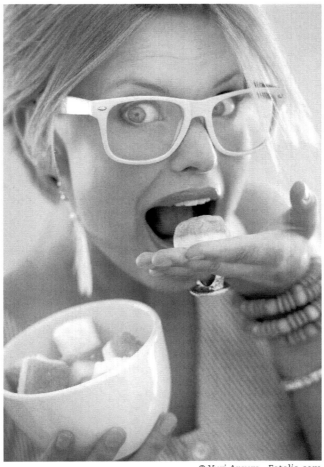

© Yuri Arcurs - Fotolia.com

Research for a link between sweet-tasting carbohydrates and food addiction that results in cravings and bingeing behaviour has been going on for many years. A 2003 study showed that sugar could act like a drug and that its effects could be blocked by a morphine-blocking agent.[21]

Consider the chilling study on rats that compared addiction to sweetness to cocaine addiction.[22] This study showed that the lure of sweetness was so compelling that rats heavily addicted to cocaine would abandon their precious white powder for sugar. In fact the cocaine-addicted rats would ignore offers of more cocaine in preference for the sweet stuff (saccharine or sugar).

The authors of the report suggested that there is an inborn sensitivity to sweet-tasting things in most mammals, which evolved because of the low carbohydrate nature of our ancestral environment. Thus in our modern sweet-laden environment, there exists in each one of us the potential to override our self-control mechanisms and lead us into carbohydrate addiction.

Heroin-like Response

Various researchers have found that high sugar diets alter opioid receptors in the areas of the brain that control food intake. The opioid family is similar to morphine/heroin and is linked to pleasure and euphoria. The more active these receptors are, the hungrier you become. This is exactly what happened to the various test subjects when they consumed meals high in fat or sugar.[23]

If You Are Addicted, Recognise it

Sometimes it helps to recognise that you are addicted to sugars and sweet tastes. If you are, then you need to consider treating your addiction in a similar way to alcohol addiction. Alcoholics stay off the bottle by avoiding alcohol. They do not give themselves occasional treats like a double scotch or a gin and tonic. Maybe you follow the same route if you suspect that you have a carb addiction?

EATING TOO MUCH? YOU FAT LAZY THING!

Do you feel guilty because you are fat?

Don't worry, you are not alone. Society has many subtle ways of punishing fat people. Somehow we have a self-righteous belief that fat people are fat because they lack the self-control that thin people have.

The World Health Organization says that we are getting fat because we don't exercise enough and we eat too much.[24] They go on to suggest that we fix this by eating less ('Limit energy intake from total fats'), and engage in regular physical exercise.

So that's it then. Fat people are weak and lazy. All they need to do is get in the gym and cut some meals and they will magically become thin.

Finding it Hard to Lose Weight?

I don't know what you have tried to do to lose weight, but I have been at it for over a quarter of a century. No one can accuse me of being slothful or gluttonous. I always followed the accepted nutritional advice and ate low-fat everything, combined with lots of grains, fruit and veggies.

I was also used to being hungry and delaying meals because limiting food intake is supposed to make one lean. I also exercised six days a week. And not easy exercise either; some weeks I cycled over 150 kilometres on the road. Surely this should have been enough exercise? The truth is that none of this worked for me.

I was the fittest fat guy in the gym! **READ MORE** My Story p. 124.

Some of this thinking is based on bad science, the kind of science that tries to imagine that the human body runs like a machine, like a car, where you put in so much petrol and you get out so many kilometres.

Which is how the calories-in, calories-out theory works. Simply reduce the calories that you take in, exercise a little more and you will become lean. If this theory worked, our gyms would be full of thin people, which they most certainly are not!

It is unbelievable that despite almost 50 years of failing to get this theory to work, so many doctors, nutritionists and scientists still believe in it. Science is supposed to be based on fact not faith, but in this case faith has prevailed. Any nationalist who counts calories and weighs meals is not working on fact but rather flying on blind faith.

The truth is that something other than overeating is making us fat.

SILLY IDEA: CALORIES IN = CALORIES OUT

'Obesity is largely due to excessive calorie intake and inactivity, not from a single ingredient in our food supply.'
Sweet Surprise: The Facts About High Fructose Corn Syrup.[25]

One of the fondest and dumbest ideas ever is that the human body works like a machine that obeys the law of thermodynamics, which says: Energy in equals Energy out. Thus if you eat too much and don't exercise enough your body stores the excess energy as fat. LOL!

Think about all the predators in the wild, how do they regulate their energy usage? Have you ever seen a fat lion? Surely the same laws that make us fat if we overeat would apply to predators in the wild? Wouldn't a lion that had a great hunting streak for a few months pick up weight from eating too many calories? Especially those lazy male lions that sleep all day while the females hunt?

Can you imagine if nature enabled predators like lions to get fat? Think how quickly the lion species would have died out if they had been overweight and too slow to chase their dinner.

As a matter of fact, how did mankind manage to get this right for over two million years, without the medical industry and the government to tell us what to do?

The First Law of Thermodynamics
Some experts expect us to believe that our bodies obey the First Law. The movement of energy is as nicely and precisely balanced as an energy experiment in a lab and the total energy in our systems remains constant.

THE DECARB DIET: GUIDE TO A LOW CARB LIFESTYLE

> 'If energy input (carbs + protein) is equal to energy output then you have balance. If energy input is exceeded by output you have obesity. If energy input is less than energy output you have anorexia. It does not take Einstein to figure this out.'
>
> Typical Misguided Internet Post

These smart scientists tell us that unless the calories you eat equal the calories you expend, you will become fat. Thus, people who get fat eat too much. If they can't lose weight it is their fault because they eat too much and are lazy. Lean people eat in moderation or are active and burn off their excess calories.

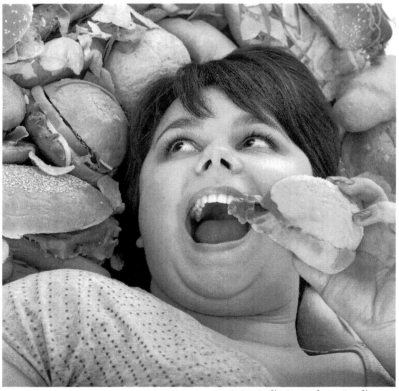

© Gennadiy Poznyakov - Fotolia.com

You are fat because you lack the character to get your bad habits under control! As Louis Newberg said, 'You get fat from your perverted appetite.'

He went on to say that 'All obese persons are alike in one fundamental respect, they literally overeat.'

Homeostasis

The hypothalamus in our brain is our built-in regulator; think of it as the conductor of the hormone orchestra in your body. It governs how much weight we can carry, whether we are human or lion. This is the mechanism that governs how tall we get, how hungry or how thirsty we are. (The hypothalamus inhibits or stimulates the pituitary gland to release hormones based on nerve impulses that it receives.)

If your hypothalamus goes awry for some reason and instructs your hormones to make you fat, you will get fat! Researchers have found that by damaging the hypothalamus of lab rats they can cause them to become ravenously hungry and then eat until they become morbidly obese.

SUGAR: SWEET SUICIDE

The consumption of sugar and sugar-containing products is so much a part of our everyday lives that it is hard to believe that only a couple of hundred years ago sugar was all but absent in our diets. Until the early 1900s, sugar was an expensive delicacy. Our grandparents and the generations before them ate fat, meat, vegetables, very few carbs and almost no sugar. As a result most of them were lean.

Sugarcane is now the world's largest crop, estimated at 1.7 billion tons in 2010.[26]

Each American consumes about 54 kg of sugar a year (according to 2005 estimates). This works out to about 35 teaspoons of sugar a day! Some analysts say the actual number is even more because the toxic High Fructose Corn Syrup is not included in these figures. (For all intents and purposes HCFS is identical to sugar, having a 45:55 ratio of glucose to fructose.)

Any sugar consumption graph you look at appears similar to the one below, which in this case is for England from 1800 to 1960. They all trend upwards, fast.

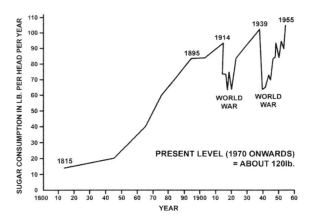

From *The Saccharine Disease* by TL Cleave 1974 – Royal Navy [27]

Some medical scientists point out how closely the rise of obesity tracks the rise of sugar consumption. Swelled by this rise, diabetes has become the world's number one health risk.[28]

The Problem With Sugar

The problem with sugar is that it is unlike any other carbohydrate in our diets. Our systems are used to dealing with small quantities of starch. Starch is made of glucose, joined together in chains. It is found naturally in vegetables, maize or wheat. Although we are used to digesting starch, nowhere in our history have we been exposed to sugar. Until the last few hundred years, that is.

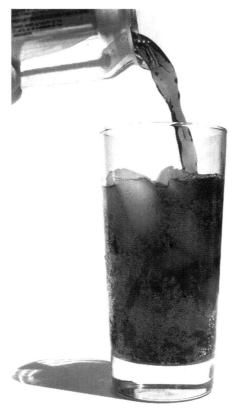

© JJAVA - Fotolia.com

It is a scary thought that most of us consume between **30 and 70 kilograms a year** of a substance which is foreign to our metabolism, a substance which is unique in its composition and its appeal to our taste buds.

There is nothing natural about sugar. It is composed of 50% glucose and 50% fructose and the fructose is the dangerous part. Nothing else in our diets contains such high levels of pure fructose. And fructose is dangerous!

READ MORE See 'Fructose is a Poison' p. 92.

Sugar Makes You Older Faster

A higher intake of sugar translates to a higher concentration of aging products in the blood. These AGEs (advanced glycation end-products) are like rust and make your skin wrinkled and your blood vessels stiff.

READ MORE See 'Why You Need to Know About AGEs' p. 98.

Digesting Sugar

Once eaten and digested, sugar gets split into its two equal parts – glucose and fructose. The fructose portion of sugar can **only** be dealt with in the liver. Once it gets there, it is converted into a form of fat called a triglyceride. A byproduct of this process is a waste product called uric acid, which is removed from the body by the kidneys.

Uric Acid

One of the worst effects of the extra uric acid is that it raises blood pressure. It does this by suppressing nitrous oxide production, which plays an important part in maintaining normal blood pressure levels. Thus, the more sugar you have in your diet, the greater the possibility you will have abnormally high blood pressure. This was exactly the finding of a recent study of almost 5,000 adolescents who drank various sweetened beverages.[29] When your kids are drinking soft drinks and fruit juices, their blood pressures are going up and so are their potential long-term heart risks.

Another problem with the extra uric acid is that it causes gout in susceptible people. A study published in 2008, which lasted 12 years with over 46,000 male participants, found a strong association between soft drink and fruit juice consumption (high sugar thus high fructose) and gout risk.[30]

A High Sugar Diet is a High Fat Diet

You can think of any high sugar drink (or food) as a high fat meal! This is nowhere near as impossible to understand as it seems. This is because all fructose in the sugar is first converted into fat by the liver before it can be used by the body. Fructose is broken down and converted into fats called triglycerides. This process is called *de novo lipogenesis*, a term that simply means 'new fat making', which is how the sugar you consume turns to fat.

These 'new fats' are then either stored in the liver as fat droplets or transported in the blood. Triglycerides end up either being used for fuel by muscles or being stored as fat. If we think of the average teenager drinking cola, the image of them slumped in front of the TV comes much more readily to mind than one of them consuming the cola after exercise – so guess where the fat in the blood is most likely to end up.

An important note: high triglyceride levels are associated with increased risk of heart disease.[31] The more sugar you eat, the higher your triglycerides will be and the higher your level of risk. Stopping or reducing sugar and refined carb intake is associated with an almost immediate drop in triglyceride levels.

Fatty Liver

Another consequence of consuming lots of sugar is the development of a fatty liver. Remember the 'new fat making' factory in your liver? This process produces triglycerides, many of which are stored in the liver as fat droplets. If enough of these fat droplets accumulate, the liver becomes enlarged and sometimes inflamed. Fatty liver disease occurs in people who consume too much alcohol as well as people who consume too much sugar. Alcohol and fructose are treated in very similar ways by the liver. NAFLD

(Non-Alcoholic Fatty Liver Disease) is a fatty liver caused by a diet high in carbohydrates and occurs in susceptible individuals. It is the most common disease in children in the USA today – it affects one in every ten children.[32]

Some people have fatty livers that you can actually see by looking at their abdomens. They will have a bulging abdomen that is quite visibly more swollen on the right hand side from just below the ribcage. When caused by fructose, this condition is often easily reversed by stopping the intake of sugar and fructose.

Your 'I'm Full' Warning Light is Broken

Another problem with the consumption of sugar is that it seems to bypass our built-in 'fullness' sensors. The feeling of having eaten enough (satiety) is an important sensation and various studies have shown that sweet drinks added to a meal have no effect on this sensation. This means that you will eat as much at a session irrespective of whether you drink soda or water.

This is a big problem. Think about it. It means that whenever you drink sweet stuff, such as fruit juice or sodas, the high energy content in these drinks makes no impact on how much food you eat.

A telling study looked at the amount of food children ate at a fast food restaurant when eating their meals with or without soda drinks. They found that the kids ate at least as much or more food when they drank sweetened soda drinks, than when they drank water.

Sugar – Just Say No

The take-home lesson is that sugar was never part of our lives and has no place in our food.

Be alert! Chefs, cooks and food manufacturers put sugar in virtually everything. You need to be aware of this and be constantly on the lookout for a sugar ambush. Just last week I ordered a cappuccino with cream, and as I took my first sip, I was hit by a rush of sweetness.

WHY

When questioned, the chef explained that he always added sugar to his cream because it tasted better that way.

Dr Robert Lustig famously published a list of all the foods at MacDonald's that do not contain sugar or High Fructose Corn Syrup. There were just seven items! [33]

- French fries
- Hash browns
- Chicken McNuggets
- Sausages
- Diet sodas
- Coffee
- Iced tea

Be careful out there!

FRUCTOSE IS A POISON

'Fructose is a poison. The fat is going down, the sugar is going up and we are all getting sick.'
Dr Robert Lustig – 2009, Pediatric Endocrinologist, UC San Francisco

Ask some nutritionists and health shop 'doctors' and they will tell you how good fructose is for you. 'Wonderful stuff,' said a health expert as we stood between the aisles packed with health products and vitamins. 'It is so much more natural and best of all it does not raise your blood sugar.'

When I told her that fructose was a poison she looked at me as if I was dangerous, deranged by the rubbish I read on the internet. But I am perfectly sane and I understand biochemistry well enough to know how dangerous fructose really is.

'Well I don't know what your issue is,' she said. 'It is natural.' Life is too short for me to explain to her, but for you dear reader, here are some facts.

Fructose Basics

- It is twice as sweet as sucrose
- It does not raise blood sugar levels (so it is supposed to be good for you)
- It is not the same as glucose
- Sugar is 50% fructose and 50% glucose

Why Fructose is a Poison

Fructose is chemically similar to alcohol and, just like alcohol, can only be dealt with by the liver. It has to be converted into useful energy by a process in the liver that produces high blood fat levels and over time creates fat droplets in the liver.

The four biggest dangers of fructose are:

1. Fructose raises blood pressure because as it is processed it results in increased levels of uric acid (which also causes gout).

2. When you drink fructose you are drinking fat. About 30% of consumed fructose ends up as fat (free fatty acids and triglycerides).

3. There is no biological feedback mechanism linking the intake of fructose to a STOP button in the brain, so that your brain can't tell you when you are full.

4. Fructose is used in cooking as a browning agent; in your body, it causes cross-linking in arteries and speeds up ageing.

Over time we have developed a sensitive mechanism for the body to control its weight. As blood sugar rises after a meal, it signals the brain to release ghrelin, a 'fullness' hormone which tells us that we have eaten enough. Fructose bypasses that system. So when we eat (and especially drink) fructose-sweetened food, our fullness meter stops working.

Fructose in Fruit

One of the main reasons why fruit is limited in the Strike Phase of the Decarb Diet is because of its fructose content, as you might guess from its name.

Mankind has always eaten extremely low doses of fructose, until we invented sugar granules and High Fructose Corn Syrup. 'But surely,' you ask, 'there must be tons of fructose in fruit and we have always eaten that?'

Fruit is relatively high in fructose but when we eat fruit the quantity of fructose we can eat is determined by the fibre in the fruit. For example, to get a similar quantity of fructose as in a can of Coke, you would have to eat four or five apples. And if you managed that, you would be full, which is exactly what does not happen when you drink a Coke.

Various studies have been done showing that drinking soft drinks bypasses satiety (fullness) mechanisms in such a way that the calories from the soft drink get **added on** to the meal, without the brain being aware of it. So you consume much more, without realising it.

Fructose Values in Fruit

Here is a list of the fructose content in various fruits, graded from highest to lowest. So if you must eat fruit, then the best place to start is from the bottom of this list!

Fruit	Approx. Fructose (grams per 100 g)
Dates	32.0
Raisins	30.0
Figs	23.0
Prunes	13.0
Grapes	8.0
Pears	6.0
Cherries	6.0
Apples	6.0
Persimmon	6.0
Blueberries	5.0
Bananas	5.0
Kiwi	4.0
Watermelon	3.5
Grapefruit	2.5
Strawberries	2.5
Blackberries	2.5
Raspberries	2.0
Oranges	2.0

Pineapples	2.0
Cantaloupe	2.0
Peaches	1.5
Nectarines	1.5
Apricots	1.0

KETONES – PRIMARY FUEL

Ketones are a normal by-product of the breakdown of fats. They are used for fuel by all body organs (some say ketones are the primary fuel). 'What about glucose?' you may ask. 'Isn't glucose supposed to be the primary source of the body's energy?' The answer is that when you are running your engine on a high carbohydrate diet, yes, then your body will predominantly use glucoseas a fuel.

However, a low carb diet will produce a state of ketosis, whereby the predominant energy source will switch to ketones.

> *'In fact, ketones are the preferred fuel for every organ and tissue, and current research shows that they are a far less damaging source of energy than glucose, far more stabilizing, less excitatory, and may, in fact, even help extend your life.'*
>
> Primal Body, Primal Mind, by Nora T. Gedgaudas [34]

Ketone Bodies

The breakdown of fatty acids by the liver results in three water-soluble compounds. Together these three compounds are called ketone bodies. Two of them, called ketones, are used as energy sources by the body. The third is acetone, a waste product, which is excreted in urine and through the breath (which can cause the famous bad breath of very low carb dieters).

Ketoacidosis

This life-threatening state is not the same as ketosis. Ketoacidosis occurs in insulin-dependent diabetics, when lack of insulin results in extremely high level of ketones and glucose in the blood. This causes the pH of the blood to become more acidic than normal, resulting in loss of water, which can lead to dehydration and the breakdown of other body systems.

MORE ABOUT INSULIN

Insulin is the hormone that regulates sugar and fat metabolism in our bodies. It is made in the pancreas by the beta cells. It is essentially an energy storage hormone.

Insulin regulates or is involved in the regulation of a number of systems. It acts to:

- lower blood sugar levels
- enhance protein creation (build muscles)
- increase fat production
- decrease fat breakdown

All mammals need insulin to survive. Insulin allows glucose to enter our body cells. We cannot survive without insulin. Before insulin was discovered in 1922 by William Banting and Charles Best, diabetics could be recognised by how thin they were. They literally wasted away.

Insulin makes us fat. Of all the hormones in the human body, insulin is alone in this effect. Almost every other hormone in our body works to increase the use of energy and thus burn fat. How fat we can get is determined by the level of insulin in our blood, and that is largely determined by how many carbohydrates we consume.

The more insulin sensitive some tissues in our body are, the more fat they can accumulate. There are few insulin sensitive cells on the backs of your hands so they will seldom get fat. Your stomach area, however, can be much more insulin sensitive and this allows you to develop belly fat. The distribution of insulin sensitive tissues varies from men to women and from person to person. Some people store fat on their buttocks and thighs, others around their middles and others in the cheeks of their face. In order to store fat, any area in the body needs to be insulin sensitive.

WHY YOU NEED TO KNOW ABOUT AGEs

AGEs (advanced glycation end-products) make you age faster. Some AGEs occur naturally and are part of the normal ageing process. Exposure to high sugar levels increases the levels of AGEs in the blood and as a result speeds up the development of various ageing processes.

The higher your average blood sugar, the faster you age.

There are two similar terms you need to distinguish: glycosylation and glycation.

Glycosylation is a normal and natural reaction that occurs when a sugar binds to either a protein or a fat under the control of various enzymes. Glycosylation happens only in certain places in the body and is strictly controlled by enzymes that are present when the reactions occur.

Glycation is an undesirable reaction that occurs when a sugar binds to either a protein or a fat without the presence and control of the enzymes. Glycation forms AGEs (which then cross-link with DNA and other protein molecules in the body. Various cells in the body, including the linings of blood vessels, smooth muscle cells and immune cells, have receptors that allow AGEs to bind to them.

AGEs that attach to these receptors, known as RAGEs (receptors for advanced glycation end-products) contribute to ageing and the speed up damage caused by age, and chronic diseases such as atherosclerosis, asthma, arthritis, myocardial infarction, nephropathy, retinopathy, periodontitis and neuropathy.

Prevention

Besides keeping your blood sugar levels low, there are a number of other ways to reduce the formation and activity of AGEs. One way is to take pyridoxamine, which has been shown to inhibit AGE formation.[35] This used to be a nutritional supplement but has been registered as a medicine in some countries.

# YOU DON'T NEED CARBS TO SURVIVE

Since time immemorial, humans have lived on a diet low in carbohydrates. It is only in recent times (the last few thousand years), with the rise of agriculture, that we have switched our diets to include a high carb content.

> *'Hunter-gatherers practiced the most successful*
> *and longest-lasting life style in human history.*
> *In contrast, we are still struggling with the mess*
> *into which agriculture has tumbled us, and it's*
> *unclear whether we can solve it.'*
>
> Jared Diamond,
> *The Worst Mistake in the History of the Human Race* [36]

Most nutritionists will tell you with absolute confidence that adults need about 120 grams of carbohydrate a day to survive, because they are taught that the brain and central nervous system burn that amount of glucose every day. However as soon as carbohydrates are restricted in the diet, the liver increases its synthesis of ketone bodies, which are then used instead of glucose by the brain and nervous system. It is in fact quite likely that ketone bodies are the preferred energy source for the brain.

Ketone bodies are made of three water-soluble compounds created by the breakdown of fatty acids by the liver.[37]

Body fat stored in fat cells is, contrary to popular belief, highly metabolically active. In a continual process, fat dissolves out of your fat cells into the bloodstream, travels around and gets reabsorbed again. When you eat carbs, they convert to glucose, which raises your blood sugar and causes the release of insulin. Insulin then blocks the natural movement of fat out of fat cells and stops you losing weight. So make every effort to avoid eating carbs.

We don't need starch and carbs to live. Remove carbs from your diet and your body will switch to its natural mode of burning fat, which it is incredibly good at, since we have been burning fats for fuel for the past two million years.

Various health authorities recommend a daily dose of carbohydrates of over 200 grams. Sometimes recommended levels go as high as 350 grams per day. This dangerous practice has come out of the drive to limit fat in our diet, in order to combat heart disease. Unfortunately the exact opposite result has been achieved.

A proper fat-burning body does not store fat and your fat deposits will melt away.

The only way we can put back the fat is by eating those carbs that turn into fat almost instantly.

THE WORLDWIDE DIABETES EPIDEMIC

What is Diabetes?

Diabetes is a disease primarily associated with abnormal levels of glucose in the blood, which leads, over time, to small blood vessel damage, resulting in heart disease, nerve degeneration, strokes and a generally diminished quality of life.

There are two major types:

- **Type I** – which is normally but not always a disease of childhood and results in sufferers having to inject insulin for the rest of their lives.
- **Type II** diabetes is much more common, affecting over 90% of diabetic patients, and is largely a disease of lifestyle. It can often be treated in its early stages by changes in diet and levels of physical activity. Unlike cancer, it is totally incurable but can be managed by lifestyle changes.

Diabetes is an enormously expensive disease to treat because it degrades and damages multiple organ systems. Thus the care of a diabetic patient can involve a number of medical specialties and various modes of supportive treatment for what is ultimately a fatal disease. Also the chronic nature of the disease clogs the world's health care systems with long-term fatally ill patients.

The American Diabetes Association (ADA) estimated the national costs of diabetes in the USA for 2002 to be $132 billion dollars. This number is expected to rise to an almost unbelievable $200 billion by 2020.

Diabetes Explosion

We are in the midst of a massive explosion of diabetes that threatens to engulf us all. Most frightening of all is the fact that some researchers suggest that the majority of cases go undiagnosed, until a related disease event brings the diabetes to the attention of health professionals.

THE DECARB DIET: GUIDE TO A LOW CARB LIFESTYLE

Below is an extract from a press release by the International Diabetes Federation. Read it carefully.

'... the disease now affects a staggering 246 million people worldwide, with 46% of all those affected in the 40-59 age group. The new data predict that the total number of people living with diabetes will skyrocket to 380 million within twenty years – if nothing is done.'

December 4, 2006, Cape Town [38]

Also, as reported by WedMD in 2010, a new study has predicted that more than half of all Americans may develop diabetes or pre-diabetes by 2020.

ACHIEVING OMEGA BALANCE IS CRITICAL FOR YOUR HEALTH

Essential Fatty Acids

Essential fatty acids are fatty acids that our body cannot manufacture. By calling them essential, we indicate that we cannot survive without them and if we don't eat them in our food, we will eventually die.

There are two essential fatty acids (EFAs):

- linoleic acid (omega-6)
- alpha-linolenic acid (omega-3)

Each of these spawns a family of fatty acids based on their original omega-6 or omega-3 parentage.

Essential fatty acids (EFAs) are converted to long-chain fatty acids called HUFAs (highly unsaturated fatty acids) and are stored in our cell membranes in the ratio we eat them. This ratio is of critical importance to our health.

Even though we need some omega-6, an excess of omega-6 is inflammatory and promotes blood clotting. Omega-3's, on the other hand, are much less inflammatory and work to enhance cell growth and repair. Omega-3's make up about 25% of the brain in the form of DHA.

Anti-inflammatory drugs like aspirin and ibuprofen work by reducing the effects of excess omega-6 release from membranes of tissues. For example, after a knee injury, membranes in the area will release omega-6's, which will cause inflammation and swelling, a necessary body reaction to initiate repair. This also causes pain which we treat by taking anti-inflammatory drugs.

The Vital Omega-6 to Omega-3 Ratio

The important thing about these EFAs is not how much of each we consume but rather the resulting ratio of 6's and 3's in the tissues of our bodies. This ratio is determined by the long-term, relative quantity of omega-3 and omega-6 we eat.

This means that we have active control over the eventual ratio of 6's to 3's in our tissues.

Historically the omega-6 to omega-3 ratio has been estimated to be 1 to 1 (or less) when we were hunter-gatherers. Today, societies eating Western diets average around 15 to 1[39] and ratios are estimated to be as high as 25 to 1 in some parts of the USA. The graph below demonstrates how the increasing percentage of omega-6 fats in the body tissues correlates with increased mortality from heart disease. The data was presented by Dr William Lands.[40]

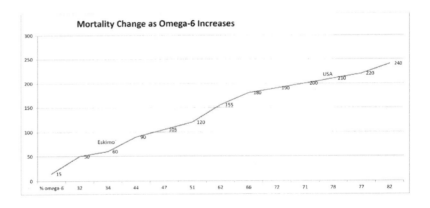

Points on the graph represent cardiac deaths per 100,000 people, ranging from around 15 per 100,000 among Greenland Inuits up to over 200 per 100,000 for Americans, plotted against percentage omega-6 saturation in tissues.

HUMAN ORIGINS AND THE PALEO DIET

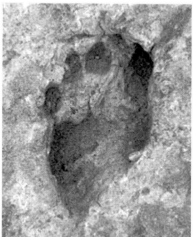

Laetoli Footprint (Tanzania) made 3.7 million years ago by distant relatives of ours. The 24 metre track was made by a small family of three walking in wet mud.

We are fundamentally hunter gatherers, sharing the same biology and physiology as our ancestors over a time span of two million years.

Over four million years ago, our earliest ancestors gave up the safety of the trees. By giving up the gripping foot of the chimp for one better suited to running, they became committed to a life on the ground. The image on the right is part of a series of footsteps preserved in the mud, made by a family of upright two-legged hominids of the Australopithecus family.

About two million years after the Laetoli footprints were made, a new species emerged. Called *Homo habilis*, this hominid had a larger brain than the earlier Australopithecines. Fossil evidence of concentrations of animal remains from this time period suggests that *Homo habilis* began to live in groups and had begun to include meat in his diet.

Then 400,000 years later (about 1.6 million years ago), a new species, *Homo erectus*, appeared. It was larger brained than its predecessors and spread out widely across Africa and parts of Asia. *Erectus* was a tool-maker and produced a wide range of stone tools, which were used for hunting animals and preparing food. *Erectus* is considered to be the first hominid to live in societies similar to those of present-day hunter-gatherers. They were bigger and much stronger than modern humans.

Homo Sapiens

The first *Homo sapiens* emerged about 250,000 years ago and a short 100,000 years later their brains were the same size as those of modern man and they were anatomically the same as well.

Early *Homo sapiens* had the ability for complex planning and used weapons for hunting. It is generally accepted that they were primarily meat eaters.

The diet of early *Homo sapiens* consisted mainly of animal protein, eggs, fish, insects and small quantities of berries and nuts. (A recent study of over 200 surviving modern hunter-gatherer societies found similar results.) Their diet was high in fat and moderately high in protein. It was also extremely low in carbohydrates.

All hunter-gatherers and predators in general eat fat for preference. They will often discard the lean portions we prize so highly these days. The Inuit of Canada prize fatty portions and feed the lean meat of their kills to their dogs.

Agriculture

Agriculture emerged about 12,000 years ago, causing profound changes in the diet of humans. In evolutionary terms, these changes have been lightning fast and our systems, developed for eating meat and low GI foods, have not had a chance to adapt to the new food supply.

Until a few hundred years ago no humans had access to sugar or refined carbohydrates and even when eating carbohydrates they were limited to small volumes of low GI carbs. As an experiment, try and get some sugar juice out of a sugarcane stalk. You will see how difficult it is to get even a little sweetness out with your teeth or by crushing it with a rock.

Endurance Hunting

There are many detractors of the theory of man as hunter of animal protein. Some say we evolved primarily eating plant and vegetable matter, yet this is unlikely as these food sources do not provide the high protein sources we needed to grow big brains. Others point out, correctly, that we are weak, thin skinned and slow moving, with only our large brains to differentiate us from other primates. Yet there is a general consensus that we once hunted and killed large, swift beasts like antelope and buck without any weapons.

How was this possible? No one was certain until a man called Louis Liebenberg from Cape Town found out.[41] In 1985, Louis sought out and lived with two groups of the last surviving hunter gatherers on the planet, the !Xo. He found them in the Kalahari Desert and lived with them for months.

He makes a point of clarifying that even in the harsh Kalahari Desert life is not a constant struggle for survival. Contrary to popular belief these people worked together and lived comfortably in their environment. An adult male would normally need to work only two or three days a week to feed his family.

Eventually they took Liebenberg on an endurance hunt. Man, as Louis found out, is evolved to run. The Bushmen showed Louis how to isolate an antelope from the herd and then how to keep chasing after it, never allowing it enough time to cool down. Men handle the heat and lack of water far better than any other animal because we have the greatest tolerance for dehydration of any animal on the planet. Thus each time the beast stops to rest, the band of persistent hunters catch up with it, forcing it to run again, until eventually it collapses.

Study of Surviving Hunter-Gatherers

An important study by Loren Cordain *et al* in 2000 looked at 229 surviving hunter-gatherer communities. They found that 'Whenever and wherever it was ecologically possible, hunter-gatherers would have consumed high amounts of animal food (45–65% of their total energy). Most (73%) hunter-gatherer societies derived > 50% (≥56–65%) of their subsistence from animal foods.' In contrast only 13.5% of these societies derived more than half (≥56–65%) of their subsistence from gathered plant foods. 'In turn, this high reliance on animal-based foods coupled with the relatively low carbohydrate content of wild plant foods produces universally characteristic macronutrient consumption ratios in which protein intakes are greater at the expense of carbohydrate.'[42]

All this shows that the human system is not designed to digest and handle carbohydrates and sugars in any significant volume, which is exactly what our modern society expects it to do. The consequence of this is the obesity and diabetes epidemic that we are living through.

Plant Life

Because of our ability to hunt and source good protein and fat, we had no real reason to eat the plant and vegetable matter that grew in abundance around us. Don't forget that plant life also knew how to take care of itself. Besides containing various toxic compounds, most plants required careful and time-consuming preparation before they could be eaten.

Once eaten, the plants offered little protein or fat to make the effort of preparation worthwhile. Even with the advent of fire-making, cooking wild plants would never have provided enough sustenance for our ancestors. So while we can be certain they ate what plants they could, plants and vegetables were not a main part of the diet until modern times.

Paleo Diets

In addition to the popular Paleo Diet by Loren Cordain, there are a number of diets and eating schemes based on the concept that we should be eating in the same way as our ancient caveman and hunter-gatherer ancestors.

The paleo theory holds that over a period of 2 million years or so, humans evolved to eat primarily meat and where available berries, fruit and nuts. This diet was essentially a low carb diet. There were of course no refined carbohydrates available as these only became available in the past 12,000 years.

A Protein and High Fat Pioneer

Dr. Vilhjalmur Stefansson was a Canadian ethnologist who lived for years with the Inuit and afterwards undertook to live on a meat-only diet for a year. He was closely studied for ill effects but there were none.

EXERCISE TO LOSE WEIGHT? IT'S NOT GOING TO WORK!

It seems so unfair. You simply can't lose weight by exercising. Surely enough, hard exercise and the willpower to reduce food intake will take off some weight, but it will come back as soon as your willpower flags.

Look around you; everywhere you look, you can see people exercising. Gyms are full. Runners are everywhere. Some cycle upon our roads and trails, while other row or mountain climb. You name it; modern people really make an effort to get fit and lean.

Are Most of the People in Your Gym Thin?

Look again and you will see that many of these exercising people are overweight. Shouldn't more of them be lean if exercise really did what it is supposed to?

Look at the explosive growth of road running in the past 30 years. The New York Marathon, for example, started in 1970 with 127 participants and by 2011 it had grown so much that there were 46,795 finishers.[43]

So when concerned politicians and health organisations tell us that we have become sedentary and lazy, preferring to watch TV or play computer games, it is quite likely that they don't know what they are talking about. A little research will quickly reveal that we are more active than ever before, and it is just not working.

Remember William Banting's *Letter on Corpulence* of 1864?[44] In it he explains that one of his doctors advised him to exercise to lose weight, which he duly did, by rowing for an hour or two every morning – only to find that although he became stronger and felt better, he picked up more weight, because he ate more.

Why Are Poor People Fat?

Now consider the poor. Around the world, poor people often constitute the most overweight segments of society. Yet many poor people make their living with their hands. They are society's workers, labouring in mines and factories, working the fields and cleaning the streets.[45]

Surely if exercise really made you thin, many more poor people would be emaciated? The key is that the poor eat more carbohydrates because cheap food always has a preponderance of carbs. And despite the hard physical work they do, they continue to get fat because of the way the carbs they eat get stored. Their physical efforts and their weight gain have little to with each other.

The More You Exercise the More You Eat

The fact is that no matter how long and hard you may exercise, your body will make sure that you eat enough to compensate for any energy you may have burned. Yes, it is possible to resist eating more after you have trained, but this is a short-term strategy. Soon enough you will start eating more to compensate for your efforts.

The simple truth is that you will always replace expended energy by eating more, and over time you cannot lose weight by exercising it off.

Exercise is Good for You

Make no mistake; exercise is undoubtedly good for you. It has many health benefits, including better cardiovascular conditioning, enhanced immune response, feelings of well-being and even possibly increased longevity. Just don't expect your exercising sessions to help you lose weight.

Exercise Keeps Weight Off

'But a growing body of science suggests that exercise does have an important role in weight loss. That role, however, is different from what many people expect and probably wish. The newest science suggests that exercise alone will not make you thin, but it may determine whether you stay thin, if you can achieve that state.'

Weighing the Evidence on Exercise – April 16, 2010 – *NY Times* [46]

Even though you cannot lose weight from exercising, it will still help you maintain your weight once you have lost it. It is quite likely that regular exercise staves off the onset of diabetes and keeps your weigh stable by reducing the insulin resistance of your muscles.

So do keep to your exercise routines!

THE HIDDEN DANGERS OF SITTING

Warning! Spending extended periods of time sitting at your desk working or long hours lounging around on your sofa will sabotage your weight-loss efforts.

Research on the weightlessness experienced by astronauts revealed that they were aging up to ten times faster when they were in space. They suffered various maladies including weight gain and sleeping disorders. (You can read more about this at http://bit.ly/18nJrTx)

As part of their research, NASA had volunteers spend up to a week in bed, in an attempt to simulate the effects of weightlessness. The volunteers soon started suffering from the same problems as those experienced by the astronauts in space, which made researchers realise that the problems were related to general inactivity.

From a physical point of view, sitting in a chair for long periods produces the same ill effects as being weightless in space. Various medical studies have shown that sitting reduces the burning of fat in the body. In fact, a number of researchers have pointed to extended sitting one of the major causes of the obesity epidemic. (By the way, a long period is an hour or more.)

Sitting All Day and Then Hitting the Gym Does Not Help

Every astronaut has exercised in space. They have used all kinds of equipment from rubber stretch bands to spin bikes and various training routines. In fact some Russian astronauts have exercised up to four hours a day. But it still does not help.

The same applies to you. Hitting the gym for an hour does not make up for sitting at your desk all day. The hour in the gym is simply not long enough to make up for all that inactivity.

Sitting, in itself, is not bad for you. The danger lies in sitting for extended periods.

THE DECARB DIET: GUIDE TO A LOW CARB LIFESTYLE

What You Can Do About it

This is the easy part.

All you have to do is to stand up once every 15 to 20 minutes.

Nothing else is required. You don't have to run up and down flights of stairs, jog on the spot or do squats. Just stand up! You can stretch or walk around your desk if you want, but that is all that is necessary.

A recent medical study showed that that standing three times an hour is better than 30 minutes in the gym. I am not for a minute suggesting that you give up exercise, I am just asking you to make a small change to your sitting habit that will speed up your weight loss and also be of benefit for your health.

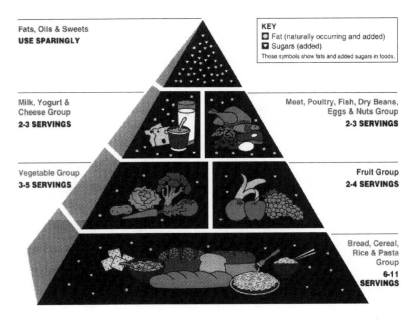

USDA *Food Guide Pyramid*, 1992

AWAY FROM HEALTH – DIETARY GOALS FOR THE UNITED STATES

In 1977 the US Select Committee on Nutrition and Human Needs released its report entitled *Dietary Goals for the United States.*[47] The document set out national nutritional goals for the people of the US and was prompted by the explosive rise of heart disease, cancer and diabetes over the previous thirty years. The committee chairman Senator George McGovern stated:

> *'Without Government and Industry commitment to good nutrition, the American people will continue to eat themselves to poor health.'*

Unfortunately, despite their best intentions, the committee made some poor recommendations, which led to a steady increase in growth of all the diseases that they intended to reduce.

Shown here is the USDA Food Guide Pyramid from 1992. It was replaced by a newer but little changed version in 2011. Its most notable recommendation from a low carb perspective is that total carbohydrate intake should make up 55-75% of a healthy diet! The guide even allows for up to 10% of daily carbs to be free sugars. The base of the pyramid shows that the grain and cereal portion should constitute about 50% of daily intake – a clear demonstration of the power of agri-business interests in the USA. (Note that the pyramid has now been replaced by the MyPlate initiative which carries almost the same information is a slightly different format.)

SPORTS DRINKS, ENERGY DRINKS – JUST SAY NO!

There are two distinct classes of new age drinks, both of which promise enhanced performance. These are sports drinks (such as Energade and Powerade, styled after the original Gatorade from the 1970s) and energy drinks, the most famous of which is Red Bull. The energy drink market was over $10 billion in 2012 in the US alone.[48]

Sports Drinks

> *'Drink early and drink a lot. By the time you are thirsty it is already too late and you have lost power.'*
>
> Unknown Cycling Coach

How many times have you heard the message that you are going to become dehydrated when you exercise? This message is driven by the commercial potential for the sales of sports drinks. Since the early days of Gatorade, we have been told that our thirst mechanism is inadequate and that we need to drink as much as possible.

What rubbish. Our thirst mechanism is perfectly capable of keeping us hydrated and it has been doing so competently for the past two million years. Humans are evolved to resist dehydration and 'dehydration is a normal physical state'.[49]

Humans are one of relatively few animals on the planet who sweat (baboons, horses, donkeys, camels and a few antelope are the others). Even among this group, humans have the greatest concentration of sweat glands. It is postulated that we lost our hair because we needed capacity to radiate heat.

We are designed to tolerate high temperatures and to perform when dehydrated. We don't need as much hydration as the adverts and sports trainers say we do!

Sports drinks are marketed at just about anyone who exercises. The higher (more expensive) end of the market focuses on the more serious athletes and athlete-wannabes. These drinks promise performance improvements, a longer time to exhaustion, electrolyte replacement, lactic acid buffers and more.

They contain high quantities of carbohydrates in various guises, but there are other downsides as well. One of these is the effect that sports drinks have on your teeth. Because most of the drinks are acidic, to prolong shelf-life, they can literally eat your teeth away. A recent study at Birmingham University showed that when a sports drink has a relatively high pH and low calcium content, it will have a high erosive potential on tooth enamel.[50]

Cost is another issue. Why pay so much for these kinds of drinks if plain water would do? And these drinks may have high salt levels (sodium and potassium), which lead to increased thirst.

Finally we have the carbs. These drinks come in various flavours but all have the potential to make you fat. Since some come in powder form and are self-mixed, carb levels are under user control. This can be a problem. If you have to have carbs while you exercise then always keep your carbs to below 4 or 5% of the total mixed volume.

Energy Drinks

Energy drinks are worse for you than sports drinks for two main reasons. Firstly, they contain added caffeine that gets delivered in a single jolt (unlike the way a coffee is sipped). This shot of caffeine is the reason why energy drinks can be marketed as 'speed in a can'; they deliver a shock strong enough to resurrect a dead horse. Secondly, they are usually taken outside the exercise environment and as a result produce a deadly sugar rush that in the absence of muscular exertion has nowhere to go except to fat stores. Energy drinks can also contain herbal supplements, taurine and other chemicals that have not been properly tested in medical trials. There are numerous reports about the dangers of consuming energy drinks in the medical literature. Medical consequences include: seizures, cardiac emergencies and abnormalities, mood alterations and diabetes. Children and young adults seem to be especially at risk.[51]

KETO-ADAPTATION FOR WEEKEND WARRIORS

You can cycle a hundred kilometres or run a marathon on water alone.

You can't do it on a whim, but once you have given your body the adaptation time to switch from carb-burning mode to fat-burning mode, you can do it. Normally this adaptation takes a month or two but it can take longer, in some cases up to a year. All you have to do is remove carbs from your diet and keep training on water.

By restricting your carb intake to below 50 grams of carbs a day, you force your body to burn fat (ketones) for fuel. As a result of the reduced carb levels, you also get decreased levels of insulin in your blood. This is the key, because insulin is the primary hormone-controlling body fat. Low insulin levels favour fat burning (oxidation) and inhibits fat storage.[52] This means your body is geared to use your own body fat as fuel and it has no need for a glucose rush from your sports drink.

When you run on fats instead of carbs, endurance events no longer become a race against your internal body stores of glycogen and glucose. When you burn fat, your energy stores are almost unlimited.

> *'... increasingly, among ultra-endurance athletes, there is greater appreciation among some of them, that they perform better when they cut way back on their carbs.'*
>
> Dr Steven Phinney, Aug 2012,
> Interview for *Me and My Diabetes* after the Western States 100 Ultra (100 mile race) was won by Tim Olson, a low carber.

Running on Carbs

When your body is used to running on carbs, the more you increase the intensity of the exercise the more carbs get burned (and the less fat gets used). This has been shown to happen by a number of studies and has been understood to mean that glucose burning is a necessity over a certain level of exercise intensity. This line of reasoning is used to justify running on carbs and to dismiss the low carb high fat diet for athletes – especially leading up to and during events.

This is not true if the athletes have been properly keto-adapted. A properly keto-adapted athlete will have a markedly increased fat burning rate and will not require the switch to glucose burning.

Benefits of Training and Performing on Ketones

When your body lacks available glucose and is in fat-burning (ketogenic) mode it uses ketones instead of fat. This gives you the following advantages:

- A steady and long-term fuel source for the endurance athlete
- Decreased lactate formation (from lower glycolysis levels)
- Lower CO^2 production when burning fat
- Better brain function (central fatigue and depression occurring late in events)
- Probably provides more endurance capability
- Probably provides faster recovery

Recovery Benefits

- Blood sugar stays low and stable – avoiding the swings produced by carb ingestion.
- There is less stress from workout sessions.
- It is possible that the lower production of free radicals from burning fat rather than burning glucose translates into faster recovery.

KETO-ADAPTATION TIME

This refers to the time required for the metabolism of a person habitually consuming a carbohydrate-rich diet to become adapted to running on ketones as a result of a switch to a low carb ketogenic diet.

A consequence of the change from running primarily on glucose to ketones is an initial period of weakness, especially for high output exertion.

Some of the earliest documentation about keto-adaptation can be found in the long-lost diary of a doctor called Frederick Schwatka who in 1878 went in search of the Franklin expedition.[53] Their party, made up of four naval people plus three Inuit families, had a month's worth of food when they left. All the navy men returned almost a year later in good health, having survived solely on hunting and fishing as the Inuit taught them.

'When first thrown wholly upon a diet of reindeer meat, it seems inadequate to properly nourish the system, and there is an apparent weakness and inability to perform severe exertive fatiguing journeys. But this soon passed in the course of two or three weeks.'

The Diary of Frederick Schwatka, 1880

Since Schwatka, a number of studies and personal accounts have highlighted this period of adaptation. Thus when you undertake a low carb diet that gets most of its energy from fat, you will have to deal with keto-adaptation at first.

Remember that most people take 2 or 3 week to adapt and that during those initial 2 or 3 weeks, it is perfectly normal for you to feel tired, listless and to lack energy. You may find that your sporting performance drops off and you may also suffer from headaches.

Be patient, it will soon go away. You will also retain or exceed your performance capabilities when you run in ketogenic mode. You can expect not to lose any performance. This is supported by a study done in 1983, using nine competitive cyclists who were confined to a ward for five weeks for testing.[54] The study found that the cyclists' sprint performance did drop off when they were first on the ketogenic diet, but returned to its previous level after about two weeks.

CARBO-LOADING IS OLD TECHNOLOGY

'I decided that what I had written in my book
The Lore of Running *was wrong.'*

Professor Tim Noakes, Dec 2012
UCT Faculty of Health Sciences Centenary Debate

For the past thirty years the belief that carbohydrate loading and in-competition refueling are essential for athletes has been carved in stone. This belief has been strengthened by volumes of medical studies, confirming how carbohydrates enhance endurance and speed. As a result, carbohydrates are the preferred fuel for athletes.

There is an entire industry built around carbohydrate-based sports drinks and performance foods. In the early 2000s the industry was estimated to generate around $15 billion per year worldwide.[55] It is probably double that by now.

Are Carbs the Only Way?

There is one flaw in all this hard work and money-making activity, however; it is based on the premise that carbohydrates are the only way that humans can achieve endurance and athletic performances.

Consider our ancestors, living for 99.99% of human existence without the benefit of energy drinks or any other performance-boosting cocktails. These people had to get up in the morning, forego the coffee and toast and get out there to forage for food. No energy bars for them. Many of these people had to track and run down game in order to eat.

As a result, the human body is adapted to getting up in the morning, taking no sustenance and getting down to the hard work of finding food. And they could repeat the exercise the next day if necessary.

The question is, how did they do it?

By using their body's fat storage, that's how. Because they were burning fat they had the capacity to keep going for days, as opposed to the few hours that they would have had burning carbs.

Many athletes have experienced the empty feeling of 'hitting the wall' during an endurance event. This happens when their body's glycogen and glucose resources are used up and they have no energy to continue. When this happens there are still plenty of energy reserves available, but the carbohydrate-trained body simply cannot access these resources quickly enough.

MY STORY

It seems that I have been fighting fat since I was born in 1956.

The first time I realised I was fat was sometime early in my junior school career, when I came in last in a sports day running race. The finishing line, which earlier had been choked with parents cheering their kids, was deserted when I crossed it. Except for my dad, who stood resolute, waiting for me to finish. There was a certain sadness in his face as he came towards me, as if he was worried for me because my fatness made me different.

My fatness remained a constant companion through my teens, easily beating acne and girls as my No. 1 teenage worry. It followed me to university, where it took seven jaw-tightening years at medical school and a couple more running around the wards as a medical houseman, to drive the fat from my belly. Briefly vanquished, my persistent foe rose again as I reached my thirties. During my first year of marriage I accumulated 30 kg of fat. The extra weight stretched and distended me, making my face unrecognisable to me the few times I managed to look in the mirror.

It took me another 10 years to regain control.

All through these years I applied my mind to understanding what was going on. In all modesty, this was no pedestrian mind, picking at articles in a dentist's waiting room. My seven years of medical training were supplemented by an insatiable urge to seek out and absorb any medical weight-loss articles. For me, the main issue was why some people put on weight so easily while others can seemingly eat as much as they want and still remain stick thin?

In my early and short years in private medical practice I ran a weight-loss clinic. And some of my patients lost weight, but in retrospect I did not really know what I was doing. I just had the old adage on my side: 'You can lose weight on any diet. It's keeping it off that really matters.'

Then during the 90s I discovered exercise and thought I had found the cure.

To put it mildly, I trained hard. I exercised at least six times a week. An average week would consist of 150 km of road cycling plus at least three hard gym sessions, where I would push weights and do spin classes. All this frenetic activity kept that fat away all right, but as soon as I slacked off, it would start growing back.

This turned me into something of a fanatic. If I had a big meal, I would be compelled to exercise as soon as possible after it to keep the fat at bay. Many times I asked myself: surely this is not the only way?

I remember when the penny dropped. As a tireless reader of articles and medical studies related to weigh loss, I read a New York Times post by a scientist who recounted his fight against fat, which began when he saw himself in his bathroom mirror as a fat, unfit, forty-year-old man. He decided to fix this with hard exercise and a year later, he was running marathons a few times a month.

A year later he found himself again at his bathroom mirror, looking at a fat, but fit, forty-year-old man.

All the exercise had made him fit but the fat remained, stubborn and unmoved by relentless hours of sweat and toil. Which brought me to the conclusion that **exercise does not work**. But I had no other answer.

Until I read the news clipping given to me by my wife in early 2012. It was about Tim Noakes and his new diet. There was a picture of Slim Tim, beaming gleefully as he held a plate laden with forbidden food including cheese, meat and fat – all the stuff I had so carefully avoided over the last twenty years. Where was the pasta and rice that Tim had advocated so often in the past?

There were seven weeks to go to my 15th Argus Cycle Tour and as usual I was seven or eight kilos over my ideal weight. From the next morning I took on Noakes' diet as a way of life.

In seven weeks I lost seven kilos and I rode the Argus that year at my lightest weight since 1998. Unfortunately I did not win! But at last I had some of the answers that I had spent 25 years looking for.

I started to follow the trail that Noakes had taken and consumed as much information as I could, which led to the Decarb Lifestyle.

FURTHER READING

If you find any of the information in the Why section interesting, you may be motivated to read further. Below are some of the books I read while designing the Decarb Program.

Sugar and Refined Carbohydrates

1. *Pure, White and Deadly*, John Yudkin, 1986
2. *The Saccharine Disease*, Thomas Cleave, 1974
3. *Wheat Belly: Lose the Wheat, Lose the Weight, and Find your Path Back to Health*, William Davis, 2011
4. *The Blood Sugar Solution*, Mark Hyman, 2010

Diet

1. *Good Calories, Bad Calories: Fats, Carbs and the Controversial Science of Diet and Health*, Gary Taubes, 2008
2. *Why We Get Fat: And What to Do About It*, Gary Taubes, 2011
3. *The Stone Age Diet*, Walter L. Voegtlin, 1975
4. *The Great Cholesterol Myth*, Stephen T. Sinatra and John Bowden, 2012
5. *Fat Chance: Beating the Odds Against Sugar, Processed Food, Obesity, and Disease*, Robert H. Lustig
6. *Low Carb Strategies You Don't Know About: 5 Little-known Low Carb Diet Hacks to Help You Lose Weight Quickly Starting Today*, Susan J. Campbell, 2012
7. *Queen of Fats: Why Omega-3s Were Removed from the Western Diet and What We Can Do to Replace Them*, Susan Allport, 2006

Diets

1. *Dr. Atkins' New Diet Revolution*, Revised Edition, Robert C. Atkins, 2002
2. *The New Atkins for a New You*, Eric Westman, Stephen Phinney and Jeff Volek, 2010

3. *The Paleo Diet: Lose Weight and Get Healthy by Eating the Foods You Were Designed to Eat*, Loren Cordain, 2010
4. *Enter the Zone: A Dietary Road Map*, Barry Sears and Bill Lawren, 1995
5. *Life Without Bread: How a Low-Carbohydrate Diet Can Save Your Life*, Christian B. Allan, 2000

Performance

1. *Challenging Beliefs*, Tim Noakes, 2012
2. *The Art and Science of Low Carbohydrate Performance*, Jeff S. Volek and Stephen D. Phinney, 2012
3. *The Paleo Diet for Athletic Performance*, Loren Cordain and Joe Friel, 2012

Other

1. *The Republican War on Science*, Chris Mooney, 2005
2. *The Hunting Apes*, Craig B. Stanford, 1999
3. *The Art of Tracking – The Origin of Science*, Louis Liebenberg, 1990

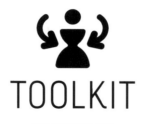

TOOLKIT

We thought of calling this section 'How'.

Under Guides and Charts you will find all the numbers for carbs in various foods, the omega balance scores of various foods, and how to interpret blood sugar levels.

The Recipes are not all strictly carb-free, but are perfect for the Stabilisation phase and your life thereafter!

The Journal pages show you how to record your progress.

GUIDES AND CHARTS

GENERAL CARB GUIDE

The lists provided here[56] give carb contents for a range of common foods. If you need more information about a food not listed here, there is a comprehensive carb listing of over 10,000 foods on the Decarb Diet website. You can search for any food by name or part of a name. Here is the link: http://www.decarbdiet.com/NutritionalIndex.aspx

Bread Products	Portion Size	Carbs (grams)
Bagel	85-100 g	40-47
Bread	1 regular slice	15-25
Bread roll	50-100 g	25-50
Breadsticks	1	15-25
Ciabatta (plain)	54-100 g	24-44
Croissant	48-100 g	20-42
Croutons 15	½ cup	15-20
English muffin	1	30
Garlic bread	1 slice	20-50
Hamburger roll, bun	1	25-35
Hot dog roll	1	25-35
Naan bread (plain)	1 small	20-60
Pita bread	large	30-45
Scones	1	30-55
Waffle (frozen type)	1	15
Wrap	small	15

TOOLKIT

Cakes	Portion Size	Carbs (grams)
Cheese cake	1 slice	25-35
Chelsea bun	1	40-60
Chocolate cake	1 slice	30-60
Doughnut (jam)	1	35-50
Doughnut (ring)	1	30-45
Fruit pie	1	35-55
Jam tart	1	20-55
Pancake	1	15-45
Swiss roll	1 slice	25-60

Cereals	Portion Size	Carbs (grams)
All Bran	1 serving	20-50
Cornflakes	1 serving	25-80
Frosted Flakes	1 serving	30-90
Muesli (no added sugar)	1 serving	30-65
Oats	half cup	30-70
Rice Crispies	1 serving	25-85
Shredded Wheat	2 biscuits	30-70
Special K	1 serving	25-75
Weetabix	1 serving	25-65

Chocolate and Sweets	Portion Size	Carbs (grams)
Crunchie	standard bar	22
Dark chocolate	30 g	15
Flake	standard bar	14

Lindt 70%	1 square	3
Lindt 85%	1 square	1
Malteasers	standard bag	23
Mars Bar	standard bar	44
Marshmallows	100 g	75
Polo Mints	1 tube (35 g)	34
Snickers	standard bar	34
Twix	standard bar	34

Crisps and Snacks	Portion Size	Carbs (grams)
Crisps (thick cut)	1 bag (32 g)	17
Crisps	1 bag (25 g)	13
Doritos	1 bag (30 g)	18
Popcorn (plain)	100 g	63
Pringles	24 g	12
Rice cakes	20 g	16

Drinks	Portion Size	Carbs (grams)
Cola	330 ml	36
Fruit juice	1 glass	10-22
Horlicks	1 sachet	22
Hot chocolate	1 sachet	20
Lemonade	330 ml	35

Fast Food	Portion Size	Carbs (grams)
Big Mac	1 burger	41
Chicken wrap	1	52

TOOLKIT

Cheeseburger	1 burger	31
French fries	medium portion	66
McFlurry	1 tub	47
Onion rings	1 portion	33
Pepperoni pizza	1 slice	35
Potato wedges	1 portion	33

Fruit	Portion Size	Carbs (grams)
Apple	medium	15-20
Apple	large	30
Applesauce – unsweetened	½ cup	15
Banana	medium	30-45
Blackberries, blueberries	1 cup	20
Cherries	12	15
Dates – dried	1	12
Fruit cocktail – canned	½ cup	15
Grapefruit	½ large	15
Grapes	15 small	15
Kiwi fruit	1 small	15
Orange	1 medium	15
Peaches – canned	½ cup	15
Pear	1 medium	20
Pineapple – diced	1 cup	20
Prunes – dried	3	15
Raisins	1 tablespoon	7

Raspberries	1 cup	15
Strawberries – fresh	1 cup halves	12
Watermelon – diced	1 cup	12

Fruit/Vegetable Juice	Portion Size	Carbs (grams)
Apple juice 100%	½ cup	15
Carrot juice	½ cup	12
Cranberry juice 100%	½ cup	12
Grape juice 100%	½ cup	15
Orange juice	½ cup	13
Tomato juice	1 cup	10

Ice Cream	Portion Size	Carbs (grams)
Ice cream	1 portion	15-35
Cornetto	1 cone	21
Fruit lolly	1	15
Magnum	1	25
Sorbet	1 portion	35

Milk and Dairy	Portion Size	Carbs (grams)
Cow's milk	100 ml	5
Milkshake	100 ml	11
Rice milk – plain	1 cup	20
Soy milk – plain	1 cup	8
Yogurt (plain)	1 cup	12
Low-fat fruit yoghurt	1 cup	15

Pasta and Rice	Portion Size	Carbs (grams)
Couscous plain	1 tablespoon	8
Lasagne (ready meal)	100 g	15
Noodles – dried (egg)	100 g	72
Pasta (dried)	100 g	73
Ravioli	100 g	38
Rice (cooked)	100 g	32

Sauce/Condiments	Portion Size	Carbs (grams)
Apple butter	1 tablespoon	7
Barbeque sauce BBQ	1 tablespoon	7
Cranberry sauce – jellied	¼ cup	25
Mayo / salad dressing – fat free	1 tablespoon	3
Fruit jam / jelly	1 tablespoon	7
Fruit spread / jam – sugar free	1 tablespoon	5
Gravy (brown) – from mix	1 cup	15
Hoisin sauce	1 tablespoon	7
Hollandaise sauce	1 tablespoon	3
Honey	1 tablespoon	7
Honey mustard	1 tablespoon	3
Ketchup	¼ cup	15
Marinara sauce	½ cup	15
Plum sauce	2 tablespoons	15

THE DECARB DIET: GUIDE TO A LOW CARB LIFESTYLE

Sugar	1 tablespoon	15
Sweet and sour sauce	3 tablespoons	15
Syrup	1 tablespoon	15
Syrup – lite	2 tablespoons	15

TOOLKIT

CARBS IN COMMON VEGETABLES

A common question is 'Can I eat vegetables?'

The answer is yes of course! You must eat vegetables, but you need to be aware that some vegetables are high in carbs and are not suitable for eating during the Strike phase.

The chart below lists the carbohydrate content of vegetables from the lowest carbs to the highest. Please make sure you know the carb content of your favourites before you start Strike.

Vegetable	Value per 100 g
Brussels sprouts	0.90
Watercress	1.29
Lettuce	2.00
Celery	2.97
Summer squash	3.11
Zucchini	3.11
Bean sprouts	3.20
Mushrooms	3.26
Endive	3.35
Radishes	3.40
Cucumber	3.63
Swiss chard	3.74
Asparagus	3.88
Spinach	3.90
Green beans	4.00
Tomatoes	4.01
Beet greens	4.33

THE DECARB DIET: GUIDE TO A LOW CARB LIFESTYLE

Chives	4.35
Radicchio	4.50
Mustard greens	4.67
Cauliflower	4.97
Cabbage	5.80
Eggplant	5.88
Jalapeno peppers	5.91
Parsley	6.33
Pumpkin raw	6.50
Broccoli	6.64
Bell peppers (red, yellow, green)	7.00
Snap beans	7.00
Turnip greens	7.13
Fennel	7.30
Kale	8.75
Dandelion greens	9.20
Onions	9.34
Snap peas	14.50
Shallots	16.80
Ginger root	17.77
Hearts of palm	25.61
Garlic	33.06

OMEGA FOOD BALANCE SCORES

Because of the work by Dr William Lands over the past twenty years, it is becoming more evident that good health requires an adequate intake of omega-3 fatty acids, one that results in an approximately equal proportion of omega-6 to omega-3 fatty acids in the membranes of the body.

The calculation of the quantity of omega-6 and omega-3 fatty acids in various foodstuffs is complex, but thanks to the work of Dr Lands there is a simple number that can be used to determine the omega balance of any foodstuff. [57]

The score is easy to use.

Remember that your goal is to increase the levels of omega-3 in your body. You do this by eating more food containing omega-3 and reducing your intake food containing omega-6 where possible.

Foods with positive omega balance values increase the omega-3 levels in your body.

Foods with negative omega balance values increase your omega-6 levels (not desirable!)

As a general guideline you can reduce your omega imbalance by reducing your consumption of the following:

- Peanut butter
- Fast foods
- Chips and buttered popcorn
- Fried, battered chicken or fish
- Margarine and vegetable shortening
- Chicken skin
- Salad dressings
- Vegetable oils

Below are some omega balance scores from the Lands and Lamoreaux article. The images give a good idea of how various common foods map out for omega balance. Items on the left are omega-3 rich (and thus 'good') and items on the right are omega-6 rich and thus 'not good' from an omega balance perspective.

Look for the balance position in the graphs below, and see how the various foodstuffs align for omega balance. The further to the right of the diagram, the worse each food fares in terms of omega balance. Note that in the third diagram, Sea Food, all the items have good balance scores; there is nothing on the bad side.

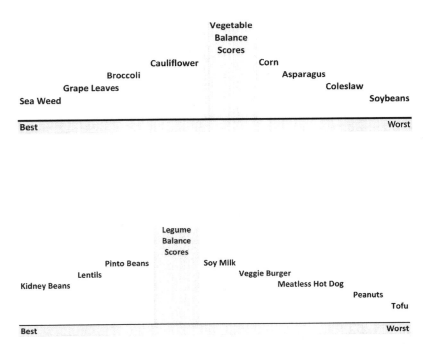

TOOLKIT

Sea Food
Balance
Scores

                                                        Crab
                                              Trout
                                  Tuna (canned)
                          Oysters
                  Herring
          Salmon
      Mackerel
Caviar
_____
Best   Good

The above values are indicative only and are designed to demonstrate the general spread of omega balance values.

The complete Omega Food Balance Scores can be found on the following web page: http://www.fastlearner.org/WebsiteFiles/FullSet 2012.pdf

Here is a short list of some common foods and their scores. Remember, the higher the score the better from the point of view of Omega Balance.

Vegetables	
Seaweed	25
Spinach	6
Cauliflower	5
Broccoli	4
Lettuce	4
Brussels sprouts	2
Squash	2
Mushrooms	0
Pumpkin	0

141

THE DECARB DIET: GUIDE TO A LOW CARB LIFESTYLE

Potatoes	0
Onions	0
Tomato sauce	-3
Sweet corn	-3
Asparagus	-4
Tomatoes, sun-dried	-4
Peppers raw	-8
Onion rings, breaded	-11
Coleslaw, home-prepared	-13
Potato salad	-21

Dairy	
Most cheese	0
Most milk	0
Most cream	0
Butter	-3
Egg	-9

Poultry	
Chicken dry	-4
Turkey fried	-7
Chicken, wing	-11

Meat	
Beef meat	-1
Beef kidney	-17
Lamb	-1
Veal	-2

Sausages	
Turkey	-4
Pork	-4
Ham	-5
Bologna, pork	-6
Salami, cooked, beef and pork	-8
Pastrami, turkey	-14

Legumes	
Beans	0
Soy	-1

Fats and Oils	
Salmon oil	263
Sardine oil	166
Cod liver oil	144
Salad dressing, fat free	0
Coconut oil	-2
Margarine, light	-8
Canola oil	-11
Duck far	-12
Salad dressing, mayonnaise, light	-16
Chicken fat, chicken	-21
Margarine, regular	-22
Vegetable shortening	-28
Salad dressing, mayonnaise, full fat	-35
Sesame oil	-46
Sunflower oil	-74
Safflower oil	-84

BLOOD SUGAR LEVELS

Despite variations between meals or the occasional consumption of carbohydrate-laden meals, blood glucose levels normally remain within a narrow range. In most humans this varies from 4.4 to 6.1 mmol/l (80 mg/dl to 110 mg/dl), except shortly after eating when the blood glucose level rises temporarily to about 7.8 mmol/l (140 mg/dl) in non-diabetics.

Blood sugar levels are usually tested in the so-called fasting state. This is when no food or drink has been consumed for at least eight hours.

The World Health Organization defines fasting blood glucose levels as follows:

- 7.0 or above = Diabetes
- Between 6.1 and 6.9 = Impaired Fasting Glucose (Pre-diabetes)
- Below 6.0 = Normal but below 5.6 is preferred

The UK National Institute for Health and Clinical Excellence (NICE) publishes recommended target blood glucose levels for people with diabetes. These are shown below, together with the International Diabetes Federation's target ranges for people without diabetes.[58]

NICE-recommended target blood glucose level ranges		
Population sector	Before meals (mmol/l)	2 hrs. after meals (mmol/l)
Non-diabetic (IDF)	4.0 to 5.9	under 7.8
Type 2 diabetes	4 to 7	under 8.5
Type 1 diabetes	4 to 7	under 9
Children with Type 1 diabetes	4 to 8	under 10

NB: There are differing opinions about the ideal blood glucose level range. You should discuss your individual needs with your healthcare team.[59]

Differences Between Measurement Techniques

The pin prick glucose meter measures capillary (small vein) blood sugar levels. The values given by this method are considered to be the same as lab test values for Fasting Blood Glucose Levels but not for two-hour levels.

Conditions That Can Affect Blood Sugar Readings

Some conditions may temporarily cause increased blood sugar readings. These include:

- Infections
- Trauma
- Stress

In such cases the test should be repeated once the condition has stabilised.

RECIPES

LOW CARB, HIGH FAT BREAKFASTS

A low-carb breakfast can be a scary experience. I mean what are you supposed to do without the cereal, fruit flavoured yoghurt and slices of toast, to say nothing of the three teaspoons of sugar in your coffee?

These recipes are really just a few ideas, which you can expand on to give yourself some variety.

Get creative! You have the opportunity to try out your own things, failing which you can always fall back on eggs. And what can't you do with eggs? You can fry, scramble, bake, mix, poach or do pretty much anything else you can think of.

Bacon and other breakfast meats and sausages are also extremely high in fat and protein; combine these with a good plate of eggs and you are set! The traditional South African breakfast of boerewors and fried eggs with tomato always works.

Here are some ideas on how to start your day.

Avo and Spinach Omelette

Omelettes are a great source of protein and fat any time of day. Try this vitamin-packed dish morning, noon, or night!

Ingredients
- 3 eggs
- 1 tablespoon extra-virgin olive oil
- Some chopped spinach leaves
- 1 tablespoon fresh basil, finely chopped
- 1 small avocado
- Freshly ground black pepper

Method

In a small mixing bowl, whisk eggs until foamy. Heat oil in a small skillet over a medium flame and add eggs. Using a rubber spatula, tilt the pan and lift the edges of the mixture to allow uncooked egg to make contact with the hot surface of pan. When eggs are almost set, place the spinach on one side, sprinkle with basil and pepper and fold in half. Reduce heat. Cover and simmer for 1 minute. Slide onto a plate and garnish with sliced avocado.

Poached Eggs with Peach Salsa

A tasty breakfast for a take-it-easy morning. A rare treat.

Make the salsa ahead of time and your only prep time becomes the time it takes to cook the eggs.

Ingredients

- 2 omega-3 enriched eggs
- Flaxseed oil
- 2 tablespoons of peach salsa (see recipe below)

Method

Bring 2 cm of water to boil in a saucepan. Rub a little flaxseed oil in the egg wells of an egg poacher. Crack eggs into the egg wells and reduce heat to a slow boil. Place the poacher in the saucepan and cover. Extra large eggs take about 7 minutes for soft yolks; medium eggs about 6 minutes. These times are valid for Johannesburg – if you live at a lower altitude they will not take as long, so you will have to experiment! Remove the egg poacher from the pan with an oven glove and free the eggs with a flexible rubber spatula. Gently transfer the eggs to a plate and smother with peach salsa.

Peach Salsa

Ingredients

- ⅓ of a cup peeled and finely chopped peaches
- ¼ cup chopped red onions
- ¼ cup chopped yellow or green peppers
- 1 tablespoon lime juice (fresh)

- 2 tablespoons of fresh coriander leaves
- Cayenne pepper to taste

Method
In a medium bowl, stir everything together. Cover and chill for up to 6 hours.

Yoghurt and Cream

This is a simple one. It requires no preparation. I personally eat this almost every morning.

Ingredients
- Full cream Greek yoghurt
- Full fat Ayrshire cream

Method
Simply mix as much cream and yoghurt as you want together and enjoy!

Berries and Cream

As above, plus berries. For treat days or when you need a slight change! Mix the yoghurt and cream and throw in a few blackberries, blueberries or raspberries.

Mini Frittatas

Frittatas are essentially the mid-point between an omelet and a quiche. If you have some spare time or it's another lazy Sunday give this recipe a whirl! (Frittatas can also be frozen, so don't be scared of making too much.) This recipe is for 24 mini frittatas.

Ingredients
- Butter or coconut butter, whichever you prefer
- 8 large eggs
- ½ cup full cream milk
- ½ teaspoon freshly ground black pepper
- ¼ teaspoon salt

- 100 grams of thinly sliced ham, chopped or other meat of your choice (optional)
- ⅓ cup freshly grated Parmesan
- 2 tablespoons chopped fresh Italian parsley leaves

Method

Preheat the oven to 190°C. Butter 2 mini muffin tins (each with 24 cups) with your butter of choice. Whisk the eggs, milk, pepper and salt in a large bowl to blend well. Stir in the ham, cheese and parsley. Fill the muffin cups almost to the top with the egg mixture. Bake until the egg mixture puffs and is just set in the centre, about 8 to 10 minutes. Using a rubber spatula, loosen the frittatas from the muffin cups and slide them onto a platter. Serve immediately.

Primal Cereal

If you miss the oatmeal that you enjoyed during your low-fat/high-fibre days, you will be so excited to try this amazing 'Primal Cereal'. It is definitely a new breakfast favorite! This bowl of breakfast goodness is smooth, warm, and creamy ... perfect for those cool mornings.

Ingredients
- ½ cup almonds, whole or slivered
- ½ cup pecans
- ½ banana (optional, large quantities of bananas are not recommended)
- ¼ tablespoon ground cinnamon
- ⅓ tablespoon salt
- ¼ cup unsweetened almond milk or coconut milk, plus more to taste

Method

Pulse all ingredients in a food processor or blender until desired consistency is reached. Depending on your preference, the hot cereal can be smooth or chunky. Warm the cereal in the microwave or on the stove until hot. Add fresh berries and more almond or coconut milk to taste.

Kickstarter Protein Shake

This shake is designed to get you going (with coffee, but you can use decaf) and keep you going through the morning (with the medium-chain fatty acids in the coconut milk). The flax seed meal adds fibre and lots of other good things, but you could also add fibre in the form of Benefiber or a similar preparation. (If you aren't a coffee fan there's a fruit shake recipe below.)

Ingredients
- 1 cup coffee, cold (you can use instant coffee and water to taste)
- 1 scoop low carb protein powder, vanilla or chocolate (remember to check the back of the box to see how much sugar is in it – there should be almost none)
- ½ cup coconut milk
- 2 tablespoons flax seed meal or substitute (see above)
- Sweetener to taste – if you really have to!
- 3-4 ice cubes

Method
Blend all ingredients together. You can do it in a shaker cup if you don't care about it being thicker or don't want to wash the blender. Drink and enjoy!

On-The-Go Fruit Shake

The medium-chain fatty acids in the coconut milk will keep you going for a long time! The flax seed meal adds fibre and lots of other good things. Make the night before or in the morning.

Ingredients
- ½ cup coconut milk
- 1 scoop low carb protein powder (remember to check the back of the box for added sugars or sweeteners), vanilla or plain
- ⅓ cup frozen berries (I used strawberries for the analysis)
- 2 tablespoons flax seed meal
- ½-1 cup water (less if you want it thicker)

Method
Put everything in the blender or a shaker cup and mix or shake.

Kat's Low-Carb Muesli

Dry Ingredients
- 500 grams almonds
- 500 grams hazelnuts
- 500 grams macadamia nuts
- 500 grams walnuts
- 150 grams linseeds
- 150 grams sunflower seeds
- 150 grams sesame seeds
- 150 grams pumpkin seeds
- 150 grams coconut (shavings or desiccated)

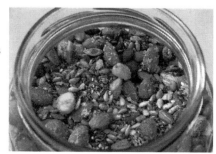

Be creative. You can put in what you like and omit what you don't like. You can also add a bit of ground cinnamon/nutmeg. If you use your own ingredients and quantities, your dry ingredients should fill a 3 litre bowl.

Wet Ingredients
- 2 teaspoons coconut oil
- 2 teaspoons butter
- 1 apple or 1 orange

Method
Mix dry ingredients in a bowl. Depending on the texture you prefer you can put all or some of the nuts in a blender. I'd recommend roughly chopping up half and leaving the rest whole.

Chop the apple up, discarding the core; or chop the orange, discarding the pips and pith. Melt the butter and coconut oil and add the fruit. Blend until smooth (I use a hand-held blender). You should have about 200 ml of liquid in total.

Pour the wet ingredients over the dry ingredients and stir well.

Make sure that all your dry ingredients are well coated. A little goes a long way if you mix it properly – be careful not to add too much liquid otherwise your muesli won't be crunchy.

Spread the ingredients over two 35 cm x 25 cm baking trays and bake in the oven at 120°C for about an hour or until roasted. Remove from the oven and allow to cool totally before placing in an airtight container.

Kat says, 'I enjoy it most with full cream yoghurt and berries or even as a dry snack.'

(Kat, who rides her bike impossible distances off-road, came home after a ride one day and found her muesli stash gone. Upon enquiry, she found her house guest had polished the lot off. When asked about it, the guest had the gumption to say, 'Wow! that muesli was good, where can I buy some more?')

Low-Carb Pancakes (serve with Berries and Cream)

I actually think these low-carb pancakes taste better than the old white flour kind and almond meal is healthier as well. Almond meal (same as almond flour) differs a bit from one batch to the next, so you may have to adjust the amount of liquid to get the thickness you want.

These are meant to be a low carb treat and definitely not something to eat every day.

Ingredients
- 1 cup almond meal
- 2 eggs
- ¼ cup water (for puffier pancakes, you can use sparkling water)
- 2 tablespoons oil (olive, avocado or coconut oil)
- ¼ teaspoon salt
- 1 tablespoon sweetener (optional)

Method
Mix ingredients together and cook as you would other pancakes.

I like to use a non-stick pan with a little oil. The only difference is that the surface of the pancake does not 'bubble' as with an ordinary pan. Flip them when the underside is brown.

LUNCH

Low-carb lunches are a lot easier to cater for than breakfasts. Most people eat a low-carb lunch without even realising it. Obviously the sandwich is out the window. But fret not! Another world of possibilities is now open to you. Instead of bread, things like lettuce and even cheese can be used to wrap up your favorite fillings, because, let's be serious, we don't eat sandwiches for the bread. We eat them for the stuff inside.

A good base idea for all lunches is some kind of meat (e.g chicken breast) together with a lump of cheese or nuts. Better yet, try experimenting with nut, meat and cheese salads topped with some olive oil.

A tip on oils and salad dressings

Olive oil and avocado oil are now your new best friends. Eating a dry or boring salad? Throw some oil on. These vastly increase both the fat content of the meal and its taste.

As far as salad dressings are concerned, you should be wary of "light" salad dressings. These are usually packed with loads of sugar to make up for having little oil. If you can't find a commercial salad dressing with low carbs, why not make your own? It's easier than it sounds. Throw your favorite spices and herbs, some mayonnaise and/or lemon juice into some oil and mix with any of various low-carb sauces.

Spicy Coconut-Fried Shrimp

This sugar-free version of classic deep-fried shrimp is tastier than its carb-loaded counterpart. It can be made as a snack, a full-fledged lunch or even a starter for dinner parties. I find it best on those lazy Sundays where you have enough time to cook a delicious lunch. There is as little as 3 grams of carbs per serving, so eat up!

Makes three servings.

Ingredients

- 500 grams large raw shrimp, peeled and deveined (thaw if frozen)
- ⅓ cup coconut flour
- ¼ teaspoon cayenne pepper, or 1 teaspoon red chilli pepper
- ¼ teaspoon black pepper
- 1 teaspoon salt
- 2 eggs
- 2 tablespoons water
- sweetener equal to one tablespoon sugar (optional)
- ½ cup shredded coconut, unsweetened
- cooking oil of your choice

Method

Mix coconut flour with the red and black peppers, and salt.

Whisk the eggs with a fork in a small dish, and mix with the 2 tablespoons water. Add sweetener if used. Put shredded coconut in a separate dish.

Put oil in a large frying-pan to about 2 cm depth. Heat to 180°C, or until the end of a wooden spoon handle dipped into the oil collects bubbles around it.

Holding shrimp by the tail, roll in coconut flour, and shake to get most of it off – you just want a thin coating. Then dip in egg, again shaking off the excess. Finally, roll in shredded coconut.

Fry the shrimp until golden on each side, about two minutes per side. I usually put each in the pan as I prepare them, but you have to watch the ones in the pan closely if you do it this way. An alternative is to coat a few at once and then put them all in the pan at the same time. Don't crowd the pan, as this lowers the temperature of the oil, which makes the contents absorb more oil and end up heavy and greasy. Tongs are the best tool for turning and removing the shrimp.

Remove from the pan to a paper towel or cooling rack. Serve with sweet and spicy dipping sauce, if desired.

Salads

Instead of lots of different salad recipes here are some ideas for each component of a salad. I have however included three of my personal favorite salads.

Lettuce: The darkest lettuces are the best; stay away from the 'iceberg' type. Spinach, rocket and darker lettuces have more nutritional value and less carbs.

Meat: Anything from chicken to bacon makes a salad simply delicious. Pan-fry chicken breasts in lemon and garlic (or peri-peri and soya sauce), cut into cubes and serve with the salad.

Garnish: Cheese is a must. Mozzarella has the least carbs of any cheese, but anything from haloumi (Greek fried cheese) to full fat cream cheese will do perfectly. Avocado is great because of its high fat content and its fresh taste. Tomato and onion are acceptable, as is cucumber. For extra flavour grind up some nuts of your choice and throw them in.

Here are a few examples.

Italian Chicken Salad

Though this isn't strictly Italian it's based on a simple Caprese salad. Use quantities of all ingredients to taste.

Ingredients
- Chicken (breast, thighs or whichever part of the chicken you like most. If it's ready-roast chicken keep the skin on!)
- Sweet rocket and crispy lettuce
- Avocado
- Tomato
- Mozzarella (I find buffalo mozzarella is the best)
- Basil pesto
- Ground walnuts (optional)
- Lemon juice (optional)
- Herbs and spices (optional)

Method

If your chicken is already cooked then just cut it into cubes or bits and cover it with basil pesto.

Otherwise fry chicken pieces in olive oil (or any other suitable oil) and add pesto to the pan while it is still hot. Cube the chicken when it has cooled. Put the lettuce and rocket into the bowl you will be eating or serving out of, then add diced avocado and tomato. Add the mozzarella. If it is buffalo mozzarella, you can cut it in circles or shape into balls and soak in balsamic vinegar. Grind the nuts into a fine sandy texture; add lemon juice and then herbs or spices of your choice. Put the chicken in the salad, and then drizzle with the nut mixture, and mix. Add olive oil, balsamic vinegar and salt and pepper to taste.

Bacon Bits Salad

This delightful little salad is like a BLT (bacon, lettuce, tomato) sandwich without the bread.

Ingredients

- Bacon (diced or cut into bits)
- Avocado
- Crispy lettuce
- Gouda or Cheddar cheese
- Tomato
- Red pepper
- Blue cheese (optional)

Method

Fry the diced bacon, or fry sliced bacon and then chop it up. Cut the cheddar or gouda into strips, or grate. (I find that a mixture of both is actually quite nice.)

Put the tomato, red pepper and lettuce in a bowl, then add the bacon and cheese. Add bits of blue cheese if you feel the salad isn't strong enough or drizzle with blue cheese dressing (this makes the salad slightly more 'Cobb-ish').

Add olive oil to taste.

Lemon Butter Prawns Salad

This one may take a little more time to make, but it is well worth it!

Ingredients
- Prawns (fresh and cleaned are best)
- Coconut oil or butter
- Lemon juice
- Eggs
- Garlic
- Your choice of salad greens
- Onion (I find white onion is best)

Method
Pan-fry the prawns in garlic and coconut oil. Add the lemon juice and any other desired herbs or spices. Hard-boil as many eggs as you feel is necessary.

Dice the onion and greens into a bowl. Dice the cooled boiled eggs, and add; then add the prawns when cooled. Drizzle the salad with the sauce left in the pan from the prawns. Add salt, pepper, olive oil or balsamic vinegar to taste.

Sesame Beef Lettuce

A low-carb Asian wrap, perfect for snack time!

Ingredients
- 2 cloves of garlic, minced
- 1 teaspoon sugar
- 2 tablespoons soy sauce
- 1 tablespoon sesame oil
- ¼ teaspoon ground ginger
- 1 teaspoon rice vinegar
- 1 tablespoon toasted sesame seeds
- Freshly ground pepper, to taste
- 500 grams flank steak

- Butter lettuce
- Shredded carrot
- Green onion, chopped
- Brown rice
- Korean dipping sauce (see recipe below)

Method

First prepare the marinade. Place the first eight ingredients in a bowl and mix well. Slice the steak, against the grain, into thin strips. Place the steak into the marinade and mix until the meat is evenly coated. Cover with plastic wrap and place in the refrigerator for 1-3 hours.

Cook the rice per instructions. Once the rice is cooked it's time to cook the beef. Heat ½ tablespoon of olive or other suitable oil in a large skillet or wok over high heat. Once the pan is **hot** add half of the beef and cook for 1-2 minutes or until lightly browned. Remove from the heat and put into a serving dish. Coat the skillet with another ½ tablespoon of oil and add the remaining beef once the pan is **hot** again. Cook for 1-2 minutes or until lightly browned.

To serve, place a bit of rice in a lettuce leaf followed by beef, carrots, and green onions. Drizzle a bit of the dipping sauce on top then fold and eat. Make sure you have plenty of napkins on hand because these are messy. Enjoy.

Korean Barbecue Dipping Sauce

Ingredients

- 2 cloves of garlic, minced
- ½ teaspoon sugar
- 3 tablespoons soy sauce
- ½ teaspoon hot chilli sauce (more if you want it spicy)
- 1 tablespoon rice vinegar
- 1 teaspoon sesame oil
- 1 tablespoon spring onion
- ½ tablespoon sesame seeds
- 1 tablespoon water

Method
Combine all ingredients together and mix well. Set aside to let the flavours mingle.

Lunch on the Go

Most of the meals described above are not time friendly or made for those of us who are always on the go. So here are some ideas for snacks.

Wraps: Just about anything can be put into a wrap and come out delicious, but obviously tortilla wraps are high in carbs. But it doesn't end there! Lettuce can be used to wrap your favorite fillings. Cheese can also be used and even meat. A common snack is cheese slices wrapped in cold meat. Prepare a few of these and you're set for lunch at the office.

Salads: Prepare a simple salad and eat at the office.

Protein plate: This is a personal favourite of mine. Boil some eggs (as many as you want) and eat alongside some cold meat or chicken. I find it best with some grated cheese on the side.

My typical plate consists of about 100 grams of biltong, 2 boiled eggs and grated mozzarella and cheddar.

DINNER

Dinner is by far the easiest low-carb meal of the day. Classics like steak and saucy seafood are the perfect dinner treat whether you're eating at home or out. Some other oddballs make dinner a real ball!

Scrumptious Butternut Soup

Ingredients
- 1 small to medium butternut squash
- 1 teaspoon olive oil
- 2 stalks celery, chopped
- 1 small onion, diced
- 1 small carrot, grated
- 1 teaspoon ground cumin
- A dash of ground chilli powder
- ⅛ teaspoon ground cloves
- 6 cups vegetable stock
- 1 teaspoon sea salt
- ¼ teaspoon freshly ground black pepper
- ½ cup full fat plain yogurt
- 2 tablespoons snipped fresh chives, or chopped parsley

Method
Preheat oven to 150°C. Cut squash in half and seed. Place the halves on a baking tray, cut side down. Bake until tender when pierced with a knife, 45 minutes to 1 hour. Scoop out flesh when cool enough to handle. Heat oil in a large saucepan over medium heat. Add celery, onion and carrot and stir to coat. Cover; reduce heat to medium-low and cook, stirring frequently, until soft, 8 to 10 minutes. Stir in the squash, cumin, chilli powder and cloves. Add stock and simmer, covered, until the vegetables are tender, 20 to 25 minutes.

Purée the soup with a blender (in batches) until smooth. (Use caution when pureeing hot liquids.) Season with salt and pepper. Garnish with a drizzle of yogurt and sprinkle of chives (or parsley).

This can be made ahead, and kept covered in the fridge for up to 3 days.

Green Chicken Breasts

These spicy chicken breasts are a great designer meal.

Ingredients
- 2 cups unsweetened almond milk
- ½ cup reduced-sodium chicken stock
- ¾ cup chopped seeded fresh green chillies
- 3 spring onions, sliced, white and green parts separated
- 3 tablespoons slivered almonds, toasted
- 1 clove garlic, thinly sliced
- ¾ teaspoon salt, divided
- 6 chicken breast fillets (about 4 ounces each)
- 1 tablespoon oil
- 2 tablespoons whipping cream (optional)
- 1 tablespoon sesame seeds, toasted

Method
Combine almond milk, broth, green chillies, spring onion whites, almonds, garlic and ¼ teaspoon salt in a medium saucepan; bring to a boil. Reduce the heat and simmer until the mixture is reduced by half, 20 to 30 minutes. Purée with a hand-held blender or in a regular blender until smooth (use caution when blending hot liquids).

Sprinkle the chicken with the remaining ½ teaspoon salt. Heat oil in a large nonstick frying pan over medium-high heat. Cook half the chicken until browned, 1 to 2 minutes per side. Transfer to a plate. Cook the remaining chicken until browned.

Put the first batch of chicken back into the pan. Pour in the sauce and cook at a low simmer, turning occasionally, until all the chicken is cooked through and tender, 4 to 7 minutes. Remove from the heat and transfer the chicken to a serving platter. Stir cream (if using) into the sauce and pour the sauce over the chicken. Sprinkle with the reserved spring onion greens and sesame seeds.

Tips
- The sauce (step 1) can be made ahead and stored, covered, in the refrigerator for up to 3 days. Reheat before serving.
- Look for almond milk near other shelf-stable or refrigerated dairy-free milks, such as soy milk and rice milk.
- To toast slivered almonds and sesame seeds, place in a small dry skillet and cook over medium-low heat, stirring constantly, until fragrant and lightly browned, 2 to 4 minutes.

Shrimp and Grits

This recipe for shrimp and 'grits' is a low-carb version of the delicious South Carolina classic. The 'grits' are made with almond meal, which you should find more filling than regular grits.

Makes three servings.

Ingredients
- 500 grams large raw shrimps, peeled, deveined (thaw if frozen)
- salt
- pepper
- ¼ teaspoon cayenne pepper, or ¼ medium hot red chilli pepper
- 2 tablespoons whisky (optional but tasty!)
- 1 cup almond meal
- 1 cup water
- Optional garnish: chopped parsley, finely chopped green onion, or chopped chives
- 1 packet sweetener, optional
- ¼ teaspoon salt
- 1 cup grated sharp white cheddar cheese
- 4 pieces thick-cut bacon
- ⅓ cup minced shallot (or onion plus one clove garlic, but it isn't as good!)
- ½ cup red pepper, chopped into small dice

Method

Sprinkle shrimp with salt, pepper, red pepper and sweetener if used. Put in refrigerator.

To make the 'grits', mix the almond meal, salt and water in a saucepan – a whisk works well for this. Bring to a boil and cook for 1-2 minutes, until the mixture thickens somewhat (it will thicken more as it cools). Remove from heat and whisk in the cheese. Let sit for a minute or until the cheese fully melts, then whisk again.

Fry the bacon, and remove from the pan. Also remove all but a tablespoon of the bacon fat.

Fry the shallot over medium-low heat, until soft but not brown. Add red pepper and sauté for 1-2 minutes, until it just begins to soften. Remove from pan.

Raise heat to medium-high. Add another tablespoon of the bacon fat to the pan and heat until a shrimp placed in the fat sizzles immediately. Add all the shrimp, and cook them for about a minute on each side.

If using whisky, take the pan off the heat and add the whisky to the pan. Stir until most of the liquid is gone, which should not take long!

Add vegetables and fried bacon to the pan and heat until the mixture is hot. Serve over 'grits', and garnish if desired.

Chicken Cordon Bleu

This stuffed chicken breast is similar to a chicken cordon bleu, which has ham and cheese inside the chicken. I've also used combinations of spinach and mozzarella, spinach and feta, feta/ mozzarella and peppadews. I've also wrapped the prepared stuffed breasts in bacon and/or spinach leaves.

Ingredients
- Boneless skinless chicken breasts – butterflied

- Thin-sliced ham (you may not need the whole slice, depending on the size of the slices and of the chicken breasts)
- Cheese that melts easily
- 1 egg
- 2 tablespoons water
- Pork rinds, cooked and ground
- Oil for frying

Method
Heat oven to 180°C.

Season the chicken with salt and pepper on both sides, and then with a herb or spice mixture on the inside surface. Greek seasoning mixtures work well, or just sprinkle on whatever sounds good to you!

Leaving about 1 cm around the outside free of fillings, layer the spinach, ham, cheese, and spinach again on top of the chicken. Roll the breast fairly tightly, and secure with either toothpicks or kitchen twine.

Begin to heat the oil in a pan – about 1 cm deep. Beat the egg lightly in a small bowl, and mix with the 2 tablespoons water.

When the oil is hot, roll the first chicken breast in the egg mixture, and then in the pork rinds to coat. Repeat with the other breast(s). Fry the chicken until golden brown on all sides and then put into the oven on a baking dish until cooked through, about 15 minutes. An instant read thermometer should read about 160°C.

Cool for 5 minutes before slicing.

Baby Back Ribs

Baby back rib recipes are usually loaded with sugar. Now you can have finger-licking baby back ribs that are just as succulent, sugar-free.

Ingredients
- Baby back ribs – however many racks you want!
- Salt and spices (see below)
- Half a can of soda water/sparkling mineral water or white wine
- Sugar-free BBQ sauce

Method
There are usually two phases to making baby back ribs – the first is a long slow braise (cooking in a little liquid) to dissolve all the connective tissue in the ribs (smoking accomplishes the same thing, I think). Otherwise they would be very tough. This can be accomplished in the oven or crock pot, but in the heat of the summer I like to keep the whole process outside. The second part is the grilling, which is relatively quick.

Sprinkle the ribs with salt, pepper, garlic powder and chilli powder. Or, if you have a special rub you like that doesn't have sugar, by all means use that. I've used Cajun and Old Bay and they are also good. Pat the spices in, and put ribs in the refrigerator for at least an hour. Wrap the ribs loosely in heavy-duty foil, but seal the sides. (If you are using the slow cooker/crock pot, skip the foil.) Pour half a can of soda water into the packet (or crock pot). (If you don't like any sweetness in your ribs, or if you prefer, white wine works well.) Seal the top of the foil packet of ribs.

Put the ribs in a covered grill with low heat (either charcoal or gas), or on a baking sheet in the oven. Cooking times for this stage: I find that 2½ hours at about 130°C works the best, but if you don't have that much time, 1½ hours at 180°C also works. In the crock pot, cook for 8 hours or so on low. Every 45-60 minutes, add liquid if necessary (it probably won't be, but the amount of juice in the ribs does vary), and turn the ribs over.

Second phase: Open the foil, or remove ribs from the crock pot, and brush the ribs with sugar-free BBQ sauce. Grill on medium to medium-high heat for 10 minutes on each side. Serve with more sauce to dunk ribs in.

TOOLKIT

SAMPLE JOURNALS

DAILY JOURNAL

Ideally you should maintain a conversation with your journal and use it daily to write down arbitrary thoughts, moods, frustrations and successes.

It may seem to be cumbersome and silly to do this but many patients have found that over a period of time, writing in your journal allows you to express and externalise issues that would not normally be dealt with as internal thoughts.

Please try and see how it works for you.

On the next page is an example. You can create something similar yourself, or make copies of the page. There is also an online version, which can be found on the website DecarbDiet.com.

THE DECARB DIET: GUIDE TO A LOW CARB LIFESTYLE

My Daily Journal

Use this journal for notes on training, state of mind, or any other relevant topic not included in the specific journals that follow.

Date	Time	Category	Notes

TOOLKIT

WEIGHT JOURNAL

You are expected to weigh yourself once a week, at the same time of day and in the same physical circumstances, using the same scale. The weekly weighing provides a clear record of your progress, which you can go back to over time.

Weekly weighing has been shown to be an important motivator as well as a key anchor for the progress of your diet.

Again you can copy the example, or use the online version.

THE DECARB DIET: GUIDE TO A LOW CARB LIFESTYLE

My Weight Journal

Date	Time	Weight	Notes

EXERCISE JOURNAL

While exercise is vital for your health and mental well-being, this program does not mandate daily or scheduled exercise. However, it is up to you to find the time to do some regular exercise. If it works for you, join a gym or a walking/running group and get moving on a regular basis.

I recommend exercise three times a week of 30 minutes or more as a good starting point. Excessive and obsessive exercising is not healthy for anyone and, as you now know, does not lead to weight loss.

Make a plan to get moving and do your thing. Try to sweat a little and get a little out of breath. And of course, log your work-outs in your Exercise Journal.

THE DECARB DIET: GUIDE TO A LOW CARB LIFESTYLE

My Exercise Journal

Date	Time	Activity	Duration hh:mm	Notes

TOOLKIT

BODY MEASUREMENTS JOURNAL

Body measurements should be taken once a month. I suggest that you start at month-end or at a recognisable milestone like the first Saturday of the month. Use whatever works for you and stick to it.

Measure the suggested body points and try to keep the place you measure from and the measurement conditions as consistent as possible.

THE DECARB DIET: GUIDE TO A LOW CARB LIFESTYLE

My Body Measurements Journal

Date	Time	Waist	Upper Arms	Chest	Hips	Thighs	Notes

It is not important exactly **where** you measure each of these values, as long as you measure in the **same place** each time. Measurements should be done monthly.

TOOLKIT

BLOOD SUGAR JOURNAL

It may be useful to measure your blood glucose (sugar) levels. It may surprise you to find out what they are. Certainly this kind of measurement is called for when you don't lose weight as expected or when you reach a sticking point in your weight loss.

As explained elsewhere in this book, it is quite easy to obtain a blood glucose tester. Learning the skill of taking a measurement is not difficult and the procedure is almost painless.

The best time to take readings is upon waking and two hours after meals.

See the section Blood Sugar Levels (under Guides and Charts in this Toolkit) for values to compare your readings to.

THE DECARB DIET: GUIDE TO A LOW CARB LIFESTYLE

My Blood Sugar Journal

Date	Time	Glucose Reading	Notes

ENDNOTES

1. Lenoir, M., Serre, F., Cantin, L. and Ahmed, S.H. (2007) Intense sweetness surpasses cocaine reward, *Plos One*, 2(8). http://bit.ly/162SqsN

2. Sweetener Consumption in the United States (2005). http://1.usa.gov/1fuVy5z

3. Nessim L. (2013 June). Scared of the sun – the global pandemic of vitamin D deficiency. http://bit.ly/16Yqp8a

4. Cordain, L., Miller, J.B., Eaton, B.S., Mann, N., Holt, S.A. and Speth, J.D. (2000). Plant-animal subsistence ratios and macronutrient energy estimations in worldwide hunter-gatherer diets. American Society for Clinical Nutrition. http://1.usa.gov/17e1afB

5. Moderate obesity takes years off life expectancy, though not as many as smoking. Medicine Research Council UK http://www.mrc.ac.uk/Newspublications/News/MRC005722

6. Lands, Bill (2008) Dietary omega-3 and omega-6 fatty acids compete in producing tissue compositions and tissue responses. National Institute of Health. http://bit.ly/1bPVn4f

7. Wikipedia. Net Carbohydrates (accessed 5 Jan 2013). http://bit.ly/GTbLTy

8. Westman, E., Phinney, S. and Volek, J. (2010) *The New Atkins for a New You: The Ultimate Diet for Shedding Weight and Feeling Great.* Simon and Schuster, New York.

9. Yudkin, J. (1986). Pure White and Deadly. Viking, London.

10. EPA (U.S. Environmental Protection Agency), (2000) (accessed 6 Feb 2013). Major Crops Grown in the United States. http://1.usa.gov/1hOeuJj

11. Marchioli, R., Barzi, F., Bomba, E., Chieffo, C., Di Gregorio, D., Di Mascio, R., Franzosi, M.G., Geraci, E., Levantesi, G., Maggioni, A.P., Mantini, L., Marfisi, R.M., Mastroguiseppe, G., Mininni, N., Nicolosi, G.L., Santini, M., Schweiger, C., Tavazzi, L., Tognoni. G., Tucci, C. and Valagussa, F. Early protection against sudden death by n-3 polyunsaturated fatty acids after myocardial infarction: Time-course analysis of the results of the Gruppo Italiano per

THE DECARB DIET: GUIDE TO A LOW CARB LIFESTYLE

lo Studio della Sopravvivenza nell'Infarto Miocardico (GISSI)-Prevenzione. http://1.usa.gov/1907F5D

12. Guerrero-Romero, F. and Rodriguez-Moran, M., (2002). Low serum magnesium levels and metabolic syndrome. *Acta Diabetol, 39*. http://1.usa.gov/1bPTUuS

13. Forrest, K.Y. and Stuhldreher, W.L. (2011). Prevalence and correlates of vitamin D deficiency in US adults. Department of Public Health and Social Work, Slippery Rock University of Pennsylvania. http://1.usa.gov/18b4etq

14. Borissova, A.M., Tankova, T., Kirilov, G., Dakovska, L. Kovacheva, R. (2003). The effect of vitamin D3 on insulin secretion and peripheral insulin sensitivity in type 2 diabetic patients. *Int J Clin Pract. (May)*. http://1.usa.gov/GTceoU

15. Inomata, S., Kadowaki, S., Yamatani, T., Fukase, M., and Fujita, T. (1986). Effect of 1 alpha (OH)-vitamin D3 on insulin secretion in diabetes mellitus. *Bone Miner, 1(3)*. http://www.ncbi.nlm.nih.gov/pubmed/3334207

16. Selye, H. (1956). *The Stress of Life*. McGraw-Hill, New York.

17. Ng, S.W., Slining, M.M. and Popkin, B.M. (2012). Use of Caloric and Noncaloric Sweeteners in US Consumer Packaged Foods: 2005-2009. *J Acad Nutr Diet. (Nov)* http://1.usa.gov/1cKZONn

18. Atkins, R. (1972). *Dr. Atkins' Diet Revolution*. Vintage/Ebury, New York.

19. Noakes, T. (2012). *Challenging Beliefs: Memoirs of a Career*. Zebra, Random House Strike, Cape Town.

20. American Heart Association. Carbohydrate Addiction. [Online] http://bit.ly/19DiOFF

21. Avena, N.M. and Hoebel, B.G. (2003). A diet promoting sugar dependency causes behavioural cross-sensitization to a low dose of amphetamine. *Neuroscience, 122(1)*. http://1.usa.gov/1gclynK

22. See Note 4.

23. Society for the Study of Ingestive Behavior (2009). High-fat, High-sugar Foods Alter Brain Receptors. http://bit.ly/GMEzwJ

24. World Heath Organization Fact Sheet: Obesity and overweight. http://bit.ly/1ajxjA5

ENDNOTES

25. Corn Refiners Association. *Sweet Surprise: The Facts about High Fructose Corn Syrup.* http://bit.ly/GTcWm7

26. Wikipedia. *Sugarcane.* http://bit.ly/GMEFo3

27. Cleave, T.L. (Peter) (1974), *The Saccharine Disease: Conditions caused by the Taking of Refined Carbohydrates such as Sugar and White Flour.* John Wright, Bristol

28. Nguyen, S., Choi, H.K., Lustig, R.H., and Hsu, C.Y. (2009). Sugar sweetened beverages, serum uric acid, and blood pressure in adolescents. *American Journal of Pediatrics, 154(6).* http://1.usa.gov/19HVWFA

29. World Health Organization. (May 2012). New data highlight increases in hypertension, diabetes incidence. http://bit.ly/1628ehc

30. Choi, H.K. and Curhan, G. (2008). Soft drinks, fructose consumption, and the risk of gout in men: Prospective cohort study. *British Medical Journal (Feb).* http://1.usa.gov/19Dcsea

31. American Heart Association. (2011 April). Triglycerides: Frequently Asked Questions. http://bit.ly/1909uzy

32. Sundaram, S. Pediatric non-alcoholic fatty liver disease. (Online) American Liver Foundation. http://bit.ly/GWtRo7

33. Lustig, R. (2009) *Sugar: The Bitter Truth* (Video Lecture – YouTube) UC Television. http://bit.ly/19wYkkO

34. Gedgaudas, Nora T. (2011) *Primal Body, Primal Mind: Beyond the Paleo Diet for Total Health and a Longer Life,* Healing Arts Press, Rochester, Vermont.

35. Unoki-Kubota, H., Yamagishi, S., Takeuchi, M., Bujo, H., Saito, Y. (2010 Sep). Pyridoxamine, an inhibitor of advanced glycation end product (AGE) formation ameliorates insulin resistance in obese, type 2 diabetic mice. Division of Applied Translational Research, Chiba University, Graduate School of Medicine, Chiba, Japan. http://1.usa.gov/GTds3C

36. Diamond, Jared (1987 May). The worst mistake in the history of the human race. *Discover Magazine,* University of California at Los Angeles, Medical School.

37. Taubes, Gary (2007), *The Diet Delusion,* Epilogue and elsewhere, Random House.

38. International Diabetes Federation, (Dec 2006) Diabetes epidemic out of control, Press release, http://www.idf.org/node/1354

39. Simopoulos, A.P. (2001), The importance of the ratio of omega-6/omega-3 essential fatty acids. The Center for Genetics, Nutrition and Health, Washington, DC. http://1.usa.gov/16Ym0lS

40. Lands, Bill (2008) Dietary omega-3 and omega-6 fatty acids compete in producing tissue compositions and tissue responses. National Institute of Health. http://bit.ly/1bPVn4f

41. Liebenberg, Louis. (1990). *The Art of Tracking – The Origin of Science*. Paperback edition, 1995, David Phillips, Cape Town

42. See Note 4.

43. Wikipedia: New York City Marathon (accessed: 18 Jan 2013) http://bit.ly/17AfcUI

44. Banting, William. (1864) *Letter on Corpulence*. Harrison, London. 4th edition (1869). http://bit.ly/16FU3Ne

45. Taubes, Gary. (2010) *Why We Get Fat: And What to Do About it*. Alfred Knopf, Random House, New York.

46. Reynolds, G. (16 April 2010) Weighing the Evidence on Exercise, *NY Times*. http://nyti.ms/19x1x3J

47. Wikipedia. United States Committee on Nutrition and Human Needs.http://bit.ly/1fuQIoQ

48. Meier, Barry. (1 Jan 2013). Energy Drinks Promise Edge, but Experts Say Proof is Scant. *NY Times*. http://nyti.ms/GMGBNz

49. See Note 19

50. Venables, I.C., Shaw. L., Jeukendrup, A.E., Roedig-Penman, A., Finke, M., Newcombe, R.G., Parry, J. and Smith, A.J. (2005 Jan) Erosive effect of a new sports drink on dental enamel during exercise. *Medicine & Science in Sports & Exercise, 37(1)* http://1.usa.gov/GTfvom

51. Seifert, S., Schaechter, J.S., Hershorin, E. and Lipshultz, S.E. (2011 March) Health effects of energy drinks on children, adolescents, and young adults, *Paediatrics, 127(3)* http://1.usa.gov/1cvYBH3

52. Volek, J. and Phinney, S. (2012) *The Art and Science of Low*

Carbohydrate Performance, Beyond Obesity LLC, Miami.

53. Schwatka, F. (ed. Stackpole, E.) (1965) *The Long Arctic Search: The Narrative of Lieutenant Frederick Schwatka, 1878-1880*, Marine Historical Association, Mystic, Connecticut.

54. Phinney, S.D., Bistrian, B.R., Wolfe, R.R. and Blackburn, G.L. (1983) The human metabolic response to chronic ketosis without caloric restriction: Physical and biochemical adaptation. *Metabolism (32)8* http://1.usa.gov/GVBb3g

55. Performance foods and drinks industry worth 12.5 billion Euros. (March 2002) http://bit.ly/1cgUfUe

56. Carb lists compiled from UMHS Adult Diabetes Education Program http://www.med.umich.edu/diabetes/education/ and from Diabetes.org.uk

57. Lands, B. and Lamoureux, E. (n.d.) Simple aspects of food help balance omega-3 and omega-6 nutrients and calories. National Institute of Alcohol Abuse and Alcoholism, NIH. http://bit.ly/GTfHUn

58. Ceriello, A., Colagiuri, S., Gerich, J. and Tuomilehto, J. (2008). Guideline for management of postmeal glucose. *Nutrition, Metabolism and Cardiovascular Diseases*, 18 (4). http://1.usa.gov/19KjMXf

59. World Health Organization. (May 2012). New data highlight increases in hypertension, diabetes incidence. http://bit.ly/1628ehc

THE DECARB DIET: GUIDE TO A LOW CARB LIFESTYLE

Printed in Great Britain
by Amazon.co.uk, Ltd.,
Marston Gate.